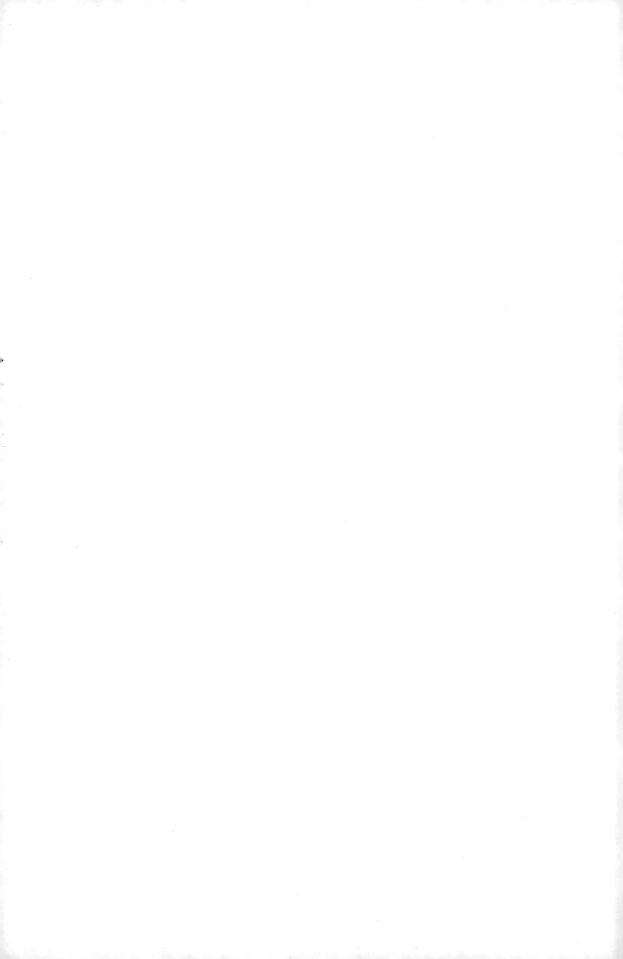

Modern Rhinoplasty and the Management of Its Complications

Editors

SHAHROKH C. BAGHERI

HUSAIN ALI KHAN

BEHNAM BOHLULI

ORAL AND MAXILLOFACIAL SURGERY CLINICS OF NORTH AMERICA

www.oralmaxsurgery.theclinics.com

Consulting Editor
RUI P. FERNANDES

February 2021 • Volume 33 • Number 1

ELSEVIER

1600 John F. Kennedy Boulevard • Suite 1800 • Philadelphia, Pennsylvania, 19103-2899

http://www.oralmaxsurgery.theclinics.com

ORAL AND MAXILLOFACIAL SURGERY CLINICS OF NORTH AMERICA Volume 33, Number 1
February 2021 ISSN 1042-3699, ISBN-13: 978-0-323-76453-7

Editor: John Vassallo; j.vassallo@elsevier.com
Developmental Editor: Laura Fisher

Oral and Maxillofacial Surgery Clinics of North America (ISSN 1042-3699) is published quarterly by Elsevier Inc., 360 Park Avenue South, New York, NY 10010-1710. Months of issue are February, May, August, and November. Business and Editorial Offices: 1600 John F. Kennedy Blvd., Suite 1800, Philadelphia, PA 19103-2899. Periodicals postage paid at New York, NY and additional mailing offices. Subscription prices are $401.00 per year for US individuals, $933.00 per year for US institutions, $100.00 per year for US students/residents, $474.00 per year for Canadian individuals, $984.00 per year for Canadian institutions, $100.00 per year for Canadian students/residents, $525.00 per year for international individuals, $984.00 per year for international institutions and $235.00 per year for international students/residents. To receive student/resident rate, orders must be accompanied by name or affiliated institution, date of term, and the *signature* of program/residency coordinator on institution letterhead. Orders will be billed at individual rate until proof of status is received. Foreign air speed delivery is included in all *Clinics* subscription prices. All prices are subject to change without notice. **POSTMASTER:** Send address changes to *Oral and Maxillofacial Surgery Clinics of North America,* Elsevier Periodicals **Customer Service, 11830 Westline Industrial Drive, St. Louis, MO 63146. Tel: 1-800-654-2452 (U.S. and Canada); 314-447-8871 (outside U.S. and Canada). Fax: 314-447-8029. E-mail: journalscustomerservice-usa@elsevier.com (for print support); journalsonlinesupport-usa@elsevier.com (for online support).**

Reprints. For copies of 100 or more, of articles in this publication, please contact the Commercial Reprints Department, Elsevier Inc., 360 Park Avenue South, New York, NY 10010-1710. Tel.: 212-633-3874; Fax: 212-633-3820; Email: reprints@elsevier.com.

Oral and Maxillofacial Surgery Clinics of North America is covered in *MEDLINE/PubMed (Index Medicus), Science Citation Index Expanded (SciSearch®), Journal Citation Reports/Science Edition,* and *Current Contents®/Clinical Medicine.*

Printed in the United States of America.

Contributors

CONSULTING EDITOR

RUI P. FERNANDES, MD, DMD, FACS, FRCS(Ed)
Clinical Professor and Chief, Division of Head and Neck Surgery, Program Director, Head and Neck Oncologic Surgery and Microvascular Reconstruction Fellowship, Departments of Oral and Maxillofacial Surgery, Neurosurgery, and Orthopaedic Surgery and Rehabilitation, University of Florida Health Science Center, University of Florida College of Medicine, Jacksonville, Florida, USA

EDITORS

SHAHROKH C. BAGHERI, MD, DMD, FACS
Georgia Oral and Facial Reconstructive Surgery, Atlanta, Georgia, USA

HUSAIN ALI KHAN, MD, DMD, MCh, FACS
Oral and Maxillofacial Surgeon/Cosmetic Surgeon, Georgia Oral and Facial

Reconstructive Surgery, Alpharetta, Georgia, USA

BEHNAM BOHLULI, DMD, FRCD(C)
Private Practice, Clinical Instructor, Oral and Maxillofacial Surgery, University of Toronto, Toronto, Ontario, Canada

AUTHORS

GHOLAMHOSEIN ADHAM, DMD
Private Practice, Rasht, Iran

BABAK AZIZZADEH, MD, FACS
Director, Center for Advanced Facial Plastic Surgery, Beverly Hills, California, USA

SHAHROKH C. BAGHERI, MD, DMD, FACS
Georgia Oral and Facial Reconstructive Surgery, Atlanta, Georgia, USA

NAGHMEH BAHRAMI, DDS, PhD
Department of Tissue Engineering and Applied Cell Sciences, School of Advanced Technologies in Medicine, Craniomaxillofacial Research Center, Tehran University of Medical Sciences, Tehran, Iran

MOHAMMAD BAYAT, DDS
Chairman, Professor, Department of Oral and Maxillofacial Surgery, Tehran University of Medical Sciences, Past President of Iranian Society of Oral and Maxillofacial Surgeons, Director of CranioMaxillofacial research center, Shariati Hospital, Tehran, Iran

PAUL BERMUDEZ, DMD, MD
Resident, Department of Oral and Maxillofacial Surgery, Case Western Reserve University, Cleveland, Ohio, USA

BEHNAM BOHLULI, DMD, FRCD(C)
Private Practice, Clinical Instructor, Oral and Maxillofacial Surgery, University of Toronto, Toronto, Ontario, Canada

CHARLES CASTIGLIONE, MD, MBA, FACS
Chief, Division of Plastic Surgery, Hartford
Hospital and Connecticut Children's Medical
Center, Clinical Professor of Surgery,
University of Connecticut School of Medicine,
Farmington, Connecticut, USA

ANGELO CUZALINA, MD, DDS
Surgeon and Fellowship Director, Tulsa
Surgical Arts, Tulsa, Oklahoma, USA

ABRAHAM MONTES DE OCA ZAVALA, DDS
Maxillofacial Surgeon, Rhino-Maxillofacial
Surgeon, Associated Professor of Oral and
Maxillofacial Surgery, UNAM León, México
Residence Program, León, Guanajuato,
México

HAMID REZA FALLAHI, DDS, OMFS
Oral and Maxillofacial Surgeon, Dental
Research Center, Research Institute of Dental
Sciences, School of Advanced Technologies in
Medicine, Shahid Beheshti University of
Medical Science, Tehran, Iran

TIRBOD FATTAHI, MD, DDS, FACS
Chair and Professor, Department of Oral and
Maxillofacial Surgery, University of Florida
College of Medicine, Jacksonville, Florida, USA

ELIE M. FERNEINI, MD, DMD, MHS, MBA, FACS, FACD
Medical Director, Beau Visage Med Spa,
Cheshire, Connecticut, USA; Associate Clinical
Professor, Department of Surgery, Frank H
Netter MD School of Medicine, Quinnipiac
University, Hamden, Connecticut, USA;
Associate Clinical Professor, Division of Oral
and Maxillofacial Surgery, University of
Connecticut, Farmington, Connecticut, USA

JAMES D. FRAME, CF, FRCS(Plast)
Consultant Plastic Surgeon, Professor of
Aesthetic Plastic Surgery, The School of
Medicine, Anglia Ruskin University,
Chelmsford, Essex, United Kingdom

SHOHREH GHASEMI, DMD
Adjunct Assistant Professor, Department of
Oral and Maxillofacial Surgery, University of
Augusta, Georgia, USA

STEVEN HALEPAS, DMD
Resident, Division of Oral and Maxillofacial
Surgery, Columbia University Irving Medical

Center, NewYork-Presbyterian, New York,
New York, USA

SEIED OMID KEYHAN, DDS, OMFS
Oral and Maxillofacial Surgeon, Delegate
Researcher, Cranio-Maxillo-Facial Research
Center for Craniofacial Reconstruction, Tehran
University of Medical Sciences, Shariati
Hospital, Tehran, Iran

HUSAIN ALI KHAN, MD, DMD, MCh, FACS
Oral and Maxillofacial Surgeon/Cosmetic
Surgeon, Georgia Oral and Facial Reconstructive
Surgery, Alpharetta, Georgia, USA

KEVIN C. LEE, DDS, MD
Resident, Division of Oral and Maxillofacial
Surgery, Columbia University Irving Medical
Center, NewYork-Presbyterian, New York,
New York, USA

GRACE LEE PENG, MD, FACS
Facial Plastic and Reconstructive Surgery,
Beverly Hills, California, USA

HASSAN MESGARI, DDS
Oral and Maxillofacial Surgeon Fellowship
Trainee of Facial Esthetic Surgery, Tehran
University of Medical Sciences,Tehran, Iran

NIMA MOHARAMNEJAD, DMD, MD, FIBCSOMS
Assistant Professor, Department of Oral and
Maxillofacial Surgery, Istanbul Aydin
University, Istanbul, Turkey

GREGORY P. MUELLER, MD, FACS
Founder and CEO of Implicitcare, Beverly Hills,
California, USA

LAURA MARCELA NAVARRO ARIAS, DDS
Oral and Maxillofacial Surgeon, Associate
Professor of Oral and Maxillofacial Surgery,
UNAM León, México Residence Program,
León, Guanajuato, México

SHAHRIAR NAZARI, MD
Private Practice, Tehran, Iran

BEHNAZ POORIAN, DDS, OMFS
Oral and Maxillofacial Surgeon, Private
Practice, Tehran, Iran

FAISAL A. QUERESHY, MD, DDS, FACS
Professor, Residency Director, Department
of Oral and Maxillofacial Surgery, Case

Western Reserve University, Cleveland, Ohio, USA

SEPIDEH SABOOREE, MD, DDS
Resident, Department of Oral and Maxillofacial Surgery, University of Florida College of Medicine, Jacksonville, Florida, USA

POUYAN SADR-ESHKEVARI, DMD, MD
Resident of Oral and Maxillofacial Surgery, School of Dentistry, University of Louisville, Louisville, Kentucky, USA

PRADEEP K. SINHA, MD, PhD
Atlanta Institute for Facial Aesthetic Surgery, Atlanta, Georgia, USA

KEITH A. SONNEVELD, DDS
FACES Fort Worth, Fort Worth, Texas, USA

OMID TOFIGHI, DMD
Private Practice, Tehran, Iran

PASQUALE G. TOLOMEO, MD, DDS
Surgical Fellow, Tulsa Surgical Arts, Tulsa, Oklahoma, USA

Contents

we explain the indications, contraindications, methods, and complications of this treatment.

Nasal Tip Deformities After Primary Rhinoplasty   111

Paul Bermudez and Faisal A. Quereshy

Nasal tip deformities after primary rhinoplasty may occur, including the formation of bossae, a pinched nasal tip, and nasal tip ischemia. Because of the central location in the midface, even minimal nasal tip deformities (small bossa) may be noticed and upsetting to the patient. This is in addition to more severe nasal tip deformities, including nasal tip ischemia, that are easily visible to any viewer. Prevention, early recognition, and, depending on the case, intervention are critical in minimizing these complications. If complications do occur, regular communication with the patient and follow-up are crucial.

Correction of Septal Perforation/Nasal Airway Repair   119

Keith A. Sonneveld and Pradeep K. Sinha

Rhinoplasty is a double-edged sword regarding the functional nasal airway; it can enhance and improve the nasal airway if done properly, and can severely compromise the nasal airway if not done properly. The composition of the nasal airway includes the internal and external nasal valves, nasal septum, and inferior turbinates. Each of these areas can be addressed by several techniques, described in the body of the text. Nasal septal perforation is another potential complication that may result from septal surgery, which has nonsurgical and surgical methods to treat, and is also described in the body of the text.

Correction of the Overly Shortened Nose   125

Grace Lee Peng and Babak Azizzadeh

The overly shortened nose can often be the result of previous rhinoplasty. The causes can include weakening or missing cartilage for nasal tip support as well as contraction and scarring of the skin. The purpose of this article is to provide the authors' approach to this deformity.

Management of the Cephalic Positioning of the Lower Lateral Cartilage in Modern Rhinoplasty: An Algorithmic Approach   131

Behnam Bohluli, Shahrokh C. Bagheri, Gholamhosein Adham, and Omid Tofighi

Cephalic positioning of lateral cruras literally means that the cartilage does not support the nasal rim. Cephalic positioning is a relatively common anatomic variant of lower lateral cartilages that shows an extremely vulnerable rhinoplasty patient. In these patients, any reductive technique, such as cephalic trimming without compensation, worsens the situation and may lead to esthetic failures and airway compromise. True cephalic malpositioning needs to be diagnosed from pseudomalpositions preoperatively. The presence of the pseudomalposition does not mean that it can be ignored. Either malposition or pseudomalposition is best diagnosed and considered in the treatment plan.

x

Contents

Cleft lip and palate patients represent one of the most challenging groups of patients for septorhinoplasty, presenting as a complex surgical obstacle for even the most seasoned surgeons. These individuals have undergone several surgeries throughout their lives, resulting in a considerable amount of scar tissue, significant asymmetries and structural deficits. Key factors in successfully treating cleft lip and palate patients are the reconstruction of the absent/asymmetric cartilages and the replacement of bony structures. The use of autogenous rib cartilage allows the surgeon to create various grafts as well as fortify the soft tissue to resist persistent soft tissue deformities.

ORAL AND MAXILLOFACIAL SURGERY CLINICS OF NORTH AMERICA

SERIES OF RELATED INTEREST

Atlas of the Oral and Maxillofacial Surgery Clinics
www.oralmaxsurgeryatlas.theclinics.com

Dental Clinics
www.dental.theclinics.com

THE CLINICS ARE NOW AVAILABLE ONLINE!
Access your subscription at:
www.theclinics.com

Preface

Modern Rhinoplasty and the Management of Its Complications

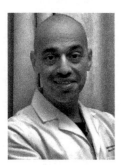
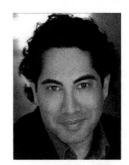
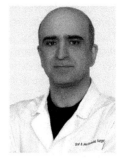

Shahrokh C. Bagheri, DMD, MD, FACS   Husain Ali Khan, MD, DMD, FACS   Behnam Bohluli, DMD, FRCD(C)

Editors

Current basic principles of surgery are ever changing. The remarkable discoveries in antisepsis, anesthesiology, physiology, and pharmacology are few dramatic changes that have forever turned surgery into a relatively safe and predictable profession. In the early part of the nineteenth century, the vast majority of surgical interventions had extremely high morbidity and mortality, such that surgery was only a last resort for life-saving interventions. There is clearly an *evolutionary force* behind the continuously changing trends and enhanced techniques that aim to improve the safety, outcome, and predictability of surgical interventions. Furthermore, the demand for less-invasive methods that are faster and safer puts additional strain on the scientific and manual capabilities of surgeons.

Rhinoplasty serves as an example of a surgical discipline that has evolved beyond many boundaries. This includes the existing broad capabilities and vast interest to perform rhinoplasty by several specialties along with new anatomically stable approaches to the procedure. Oral and maxillofacial surgeons (OMS) are relatively new in this arena. Only a handful of OMS acquired this advanced skill from cross-specialty colleagues in the late 1980s and subsequently produced very minimal contributions to the scientific literature on the topic. However, in the last several years, a large variety of peer-reviewed articles and text with major contributions by OMS have been published. The profession has embraced this field, although generally requiring postresidency fellowship training to achieve acceptable surgical competence. In fact, the modern approach to rhinoplasty is more "maxillofacial" than ever before. Initial techniques of reductive rhinoplasty were based on basic changes in the more superficial anatomic bony and cartilaginous structures. This limited approach resulted in many reconstructive chal-

Oral Maxillofacial Surg Clin N Am 33 (2021) xiii–xiv
https://doi.org/10.1016/j.coms.2020.09.009
1042-3699/21/© 2020 Published by Elsevier Inc.

lenges and long-term unstable results. The next major evolutionary change was the application of grafts to change and construct of the nose in 3 dimensions while preserving function. Today, the concept of preservation rhinoplasty is the culmination of grafting and skeletal changes in the nasomaxillary and cartilaginous anatomy. This conceptual approach addresses deeper maxillofacial anatomic layers, aiming to provide more lasting and predictable results.

This issue of *Oral and Maxillofacial Surgery Clinics* is a significant step forward for our specialty and complements our prior February 2012 *Oral and Maxillofacial Surgery Clinics* issue on Rhinoplasty: Current Therapy. Our profession and specialty have to further evolve beyond just previously established techniques and embrace modern developments. Furthermore, recognition and addressing unwanted cosmetic and functional outcomes must be an integral part of our subspecialty development. The aim of this issue is to familiarize our readers with recent developments that are continuing to change this field and to maintain our specialty at the forefront of Modern Rhinoplasty and the Management of Its Complications.

Shahrokh C. Bagheri, DMD, MD, FACS
Georgia Oral and Facial Reconstructive Surgery
4561 Olde Perimeter Way
Atlanta, GA 30346, USA

Husain Ali Khan, MD, DMD, FACS
Georgia Oral and Facial Reconstructive Surgery
11975 Morris Road
Suite 220
Alpharetta, GA 30005, USA

Behnam Bohluli, DMD, FRCD(C)
Department of Oral and Maxillofacial Surgery
University of Toronto
124 Edward Street
Toronto ON M5G 1G6, Canada

E-mail addresses:
sbagher@hotmail.com (S.C. Bagheri)
husainakmd@yahoo.com (H.A. Khan)
bbohluli@yahoo.com (B. Bohluli)

New Horizons in Imaging and Diagnosis in Rhinoplasty

Gregory P. Mueller, MD[a], Husain Ali Khan, MD, DMD, MCh[b,*],
James D. Frame, CF, FRCS(Plast)[c]

KEYWORDS

• Cone beam computed tomography • Rhinoplasty • Three-dimensional

KEY POINTS

• Maxillofacial 3D CT imaging allows precise skeletal evaluation for rhinoplasty.
• Three-dimensional photography enhances appreciation of pre- and post-operative assessments.
• Pre- and post-operative photo documentation remains the standard for any facial cosmetic surgery.

THREE-DIMENSIONAL IMAGING IN RHINOPLASTY

Three-dimensional (3D) surface imaging has found its place in aesthetic surgery globally. The first attempt to use 3D surface imaging technique in clinic was in 1944 by Thalmaan,[1] who used stereo photogrammetry to examine an adult with facial asymmetry and a baby with Pierre Robin syndrome.

Early studies involving 3D surface imaging systems were mainly completed by using stereo photogrammetry. Although the results were not precise enough and hard to be quantitative, it still showed that 3D surface imaging system did have great potentials and apparent superiority compared with 2D photography. Other techniques such as Moiré topography,[2,3] laser scanning,[4–10] structured light, and so on have been developed and studied. As a result of the various studies of 3D imaging, it is apparent that the technology is best used to determine objective changes in volume such as in breast surgery and fat injections. The static 3D image capture provides accurate objective true surface dimensions, morphologic changes, and volumetric changes when comparing before and after results. Another very valuable use of the 3D technology is to be able to show prospective patients how they may look with various procedures and also to allow breast implant patients the ability to participate in the selection of breast implant sizes. In patients who desire a change in the appearance of the nose, the surgeon can use software-morphing tools to change the shape and contours of the nose, thus allowing each patient to understand the realistic goals of a rhinoplasty.

Using oVio360 dynamic imaging in nasal surgery allows the patient and surgeon to observe and document movement of the nasal tip with animation (Figs. 1–3). Thus, when comparing the before and after dynamic images, the surgeon will be able to document correction of issues such as a plunging tip. Regardless of whether a static image or dynamic is captured, it is important to have a comprehensive digital record of the morphologic features of the nose so that operative planning can be completed and the ultimate result can be recorded and reviewed with each patient. The oVio360 images are used in all steps of the patient experience including the initial consultation, preoperative visit, intraoperative guidance, and

a Private Practice, 436 N Bedford Drive, Suite 212, Beverly Hills, California, USA; b Georgia Oral and Facial Reconstructive Surgery, 11975 Morris Road, Suite 220, Alpharetta, GA 30005, USA; c The School of Medicine, Anglia Ruskin University, Chelmsford, Essex, UK
* Corresponding author.
E-mail address: husainakmd@yahoo.com

Oral Maxillofacial Surg Clin N Am 33 (2021) 1–5
https://doi.org/10.1016/j.coms.2020.09.014
1042-3699/21/© 2020 Elsevier Inc. All rights reserved.

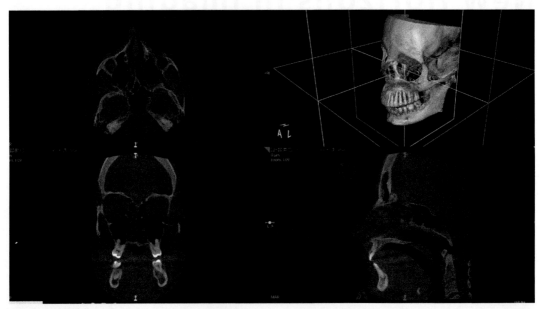

Fig. 1. CBCT analysis of of the cranio-maxillofacial region displaying the transverse (top left), sagittal (bottom right), and coronal (bottom left) views along with the 3D reconstruction (top right).

postoperative follow-up and for presentation and publication. Being able to show actual before and after images gives each prospective patient the opportunity to understand the surgeon's results and aesthetic ideal.

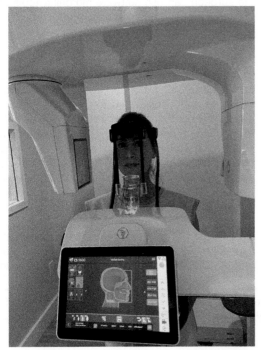

Fig. 2. Patient positioned in the CBCT device for a scan.

Currently, most surgeons performing rhinoplasty procedures use 2D photography to evaluate new patients, to document results, and to plan a successful procedure. Two-dimensional photography lacks the ability to document the entire clinical picture. In today's cosmetic medicine market, it is more important than ever before to document results from various procedures such as rhinoplasty.

Being able to illustrate a complete clinical condition with 360-degree dynamic imaging and/or 3D capture enables surgeons to communicate with patients more clearly and to also develop a surgical plan that will be successful. Evaluation of results is also much more comprehensive with a complete clinical picture of outcomes obtained with rhinoplasty. For a surgeon, the ability to go back and review a complete lifelike before image of the face and nose compared with the results provides such important lessons of learning. In addition, with today's savvy consumers, it is more important than ever to be able to provide patients with state-of-the-art imaging that is better than the pictures that one can capture on any smart phone. Being able to sit down with each patient and review a high-quality 3D digital capture is an essential tool for today's successful rhinoplasty surgeon. New technology that results in 360-degree motion capture with the oVio360 Dynamic Imaging System is also being introduced to the market. This new system allows perfectly standardized images to be captured before and after

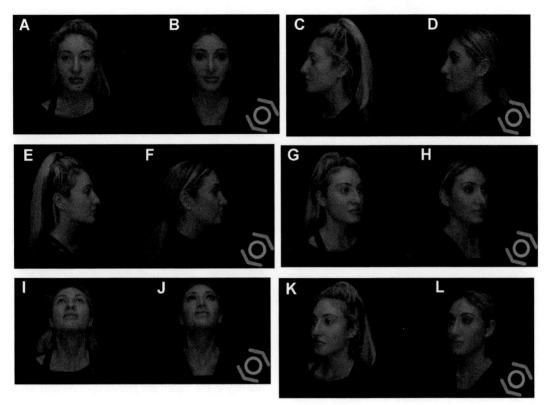

Fig. 3. Standard photography for rhinoplasty surgery.

all procedures. Using the unique self-centering technology, images are easily obtained and always perfectly positioned and lighted for standardization. Regarding the face and nose, the workflow and capture of oVio360 images includes 5 views: (1) repose, (2) smile/animation, (3) chin up, (4) chin down, and (5) relaxation and flexion of the neck muscles (**Box 1**). Each 360-degree view capture takes 12 seconds, and the resultant digital file provides a complete picture of the shape and form of the head and neck as well as nerve and muscle function. Being able to capture the face and body in motion provides the most lifelike capture of the face and body. Dynamic imaging allows the understanding of skin quality, muscle, and nerve function. Visualizing the nose and face in animation allows one to see themselves exactly as others view them. With this process, the provider and the patient have a comprehensive lifelike digital medical record that will capture all perspectives of each therapeutic intervention. With today's advanced technology that addresses all aspects of the skin and underlying soft tissue, motion capture is the only imaging technology that captures the complete clinical picture.

The differences between 2D imaging and 3D capture are significant. Standard photographs

only provide a limited view of the anatomy. Being able to determine the depth and shape of the face and nose is limited and the ability to rotate and view the nose is not possible. With 3D surface

---

Box 1
oVio360 dynamic imaging workflow for face and nose

Workflow Image Capture 360 Degree Revolution

1. Repose: physical shape and form of the nose and the entire surrounding facial and neck anatomy

2. Smile/animation: nasal movement with animation, that is, plunging tip, flaring nostrils etc., nerve and muscle functionality, skin turgor, dynamic rhytids

3. Chin up: worm's eye view of nose, nostril shape, symmetry etc.

4. Chin down: nasal dorsum, bony pyramid

5. Neck muscle flexion and relaxation: lip complex movement and symmetry, evaluation of motor nerve and muscle functionality of remainder of head and neck

imaging, the subject can be viewed in all perspectives and a true lifelike image with skin texture and x, y, and z coordinates is created. In cases of significant deformity such as trauma or congenital defects, an MRI/computed axial tomography scan (CAT) scan can be used to document the internal structures of the nose, sinuses, facial bones etc. Software has been developed to combine the results of the 3D surface imaging with the MRI/CAT scan to provide a complete 3D model of the surface and underlying subcutaneous and bony anatomy. This type of combined imaging is used in complex rhinoplasty/facial procedures that involve deformities that may be congenital (cleft deformities) and/or posttraumatic or procedures involving deeper structures including cartilage, bone, and mucosal soft tissue.

CHOOSING IMAGING TECHNOLOGY FOR RHINOPLASTY

Documentation of results in plastic surgery is most accurately recorded with photographs, 3D imaging, or dynamic motion capture. Before and after images have become the gold standard in plastic surgery, with 3D imaging and dynamic imaging being the most comprehensive technology to capture the true shape and form of the nose and surrounding facial structures. Written descriptions of the before and after appearance of the nose and face would be extremely time consuming and is not practical. A comparison of oVio360 Imaging with 2 popular 3D technologies illustrates the value of each imaging approach (**Table 1**).

When considering any new device, one must always consider cost, ease of use, and profitability. Imaging devices are harder to rationalize costs, as one cannot see the direct profitability of the technology. In today's market, the need to provide exceptional results is more important than ever. The ability to communicate with images is very helpful in the consultation process. Therefore, it is important to understand the importance of making an investment in imaging technology that will serve as a tremendous valuable communication tool in the consultation process, to plan surgery and to evaluate results.

Cone Beam Computed Tomography

The cone beam computed tomography (CBCT) scan has established it place well in Oral and Maxillofacial Surgery, as a valuable tool to aid in the diagnosis and treatment planning of both dentoalveolar and craniomaxillofacial procedures. It has also been an essential tool in treatment planning for orthognathic surgery.

Modern rhinoplasty has also advanced with development of preservation rhinoplasty.

CBCT scans are now been used in greater frequency in the treatment planning of rhinoplasty.

Cone beam computed tomography evaluation in rhinoplasty

Nasal bones: The length and angulation of the nasal bones can be visualized clearly in both lateral and frontal views. This is of particular importance in letdown techniques in preservation rhinoplasty.

Table 1
Comparison of 3 imaging technologies

Imaging Devices	oVio360 Dynamic Imaging	Canfield 3D	Crisalix
Advantages	Dynamic 360 Capture True before and after images, easy capture, self-centering/ positioning technology, lifelike dynamic capture	3D capture with morphing capabilities, measurement of changes	3D capture with morphing capabilities measurement of changes
Disadvantages	No 3D morphing	Works best with breast/volumetric changes	Works best with breast/volumetric changes
Scanning potential	Entire head, body, and extremities	Head and body	Head and body
Limitations	Size of device	Size of device, ability to capture standardized comparative images is technician dependent, circumferential head is not imaged	Ability to capture before and after comparison views is technician dependent, circumferential head is not imaged

Septum: The CBCT evaluation of both the cartilaginous and bony septum gives the surgeon an accurate view of the bony and cartilaginous septum. This is especially important in complex septal procedures that require correction of deviations and in preservation of rhinoplasty techniques. It gives the surgeon additional information to accurately plan the cartilaginous septal incisions as well as osteotomies.

Turbinates: The CBCT scan is useful for evaluation of the size, shape, and possible pathology.

Bony aperture: Preoperative analysis indicates that a wide variation exists in lateral nasal wall anatomy and angulation; the CBCT scan gives an accurate analysis of these anatomic variations.

SUMMARY

The CBCT scan is a well-established diagnostic tool in oral and maxillofacial surgery; it can be a practical diagnostic tool for all surgeons performing rhinoplasty. Three-dimensional photography is becoming more common allowing for a more dynamic facial evaluation, although it is associated with increased cost.

DISCLOSURE

The authors have nothing to disclose.

REFERENCES

1. Thalmaan D. Die Stereogrammetrie: ein diagnostisches Hilfsmittel in der Kieferorthopaedie [Stereophotogrammetry: a diagnostic device in orthodontology]. Zurich (Switzerland): University Zurich; 1944.
2. Douglas MS, Gonzalez R Jr. Moiré topography of the face: its application in mea- suring soft tissue asymmetries. Am J Orthod 1986;89:177.
3. Kawano Y. Three dimensional analysis of the face in respect of zygomatic fractures and evaluation of the surgery with the aid of Moiré topography. J Craniomaxillofac Surg 1987;15:68–74.
4. Aung S, Ngim R, Lee S. Evaluation of the laser scanner as a surface measuring tool and its accuracy compared with direct facial anthropometric measurements. Br J Plast Surg 1995;48:551–8.
5. Kovacs L, Zimmermann A, Brockmann G, et al. Three-dimensional recording of the human face with a 3D laser scanner. J Plast Reconstr Aesthet Surg 2006;59:1193–202.
6. Zhe-yuan Y, Xiong-zheng M, Jia-qi Z, et al. The clinical operational experience of single-shot three-dimensional laser scanning on 3-D craniofacial surface images. Chin J Aesthet Med 2007.
7. Kovacs L, Zimmermann A, Brockmann G, et al. Accuracy and precision of the three-dimensional assessment of the facial surface using a 3-D laser scanner. IEEE Trans Med Imaging 2006;25:742–54.
8. Li Y, Yang X, Li D. The Application of Three-Dimensional Surface Imaging System in Plastic and Reconstructive Surgery. Ann Plast Surg 2016;77:S76–83.
9. Jamal J. Three-dimensional surface imaging in plastic surgery. Biomed J Sci Tech Res 2018;4(3).
10. Tzou C, Frey M. Evolution of 3D Surface Imaging Systems in Facial Plastic Surgery. Facial Plast Surg Clin North Am 2011;19:591–602.

Preservation Rhinoplasty for the Dorsum and Tip

Abraham Montes de Oca Zavala, DDS*, Laura Marcela Navarro Arias, DDS[1]

KEYWORDS

- Preservation rhinoplasty • Low septal strip • Posterior strut • Dorsum preservation
- Tip preservation • Columellar strut

KEY POINTS

- The main purpose of preservation rhinoplasty is to maintain cartilages, ligaments, and the osseo-cartilaginous dorsum to provide the patient with natural aesthetic and functional results.
- This new approach marks a change from both resection and structural rhinoplasty and is leading to a new terminology, "preservation rhinoplasty."
- In the authors' technique, the posterior strut can be used to change the final position and projection of the tip and modify the length and angle of the columella.

The main purpose of this innovating surgical technique is the preservation of the nasal cartilages, ligaments, and the osseocartilaginous dorsum by performing an elevation of the skin in a subperichondrial and subperiosteal plane. If the preexisting nasal dorsum can be kept intact, then it is possible to preserve the natural aesthetic dorsum as well as nasal function. In addition, one can avoid many of the secondary deformities that lead to revision surgery.[1]

Preservation rhinoplasty has some principles that keep the philosophy of "less is more":

1. Elevating the skin sleeve in a subperichondrial or subperiosteal dissection plane
2. Preservation of osseocartilaginous dorsum
3. Maintaining cartilages
4. Maintaining ligaments
5. Achieving natural and aesthetic dorsal lines

To achieve these statements, the surgeon must have advanced surgical skills as well as a knowledge of the surgical anatomy and the variations of the preservation rhinoplasty techniques for the dorsum and the tip.

The goal is to replace resection with preservation, excision with manipulation, and secondary rib reconstruction with minimal revisions. In summary, this new approach marks a change from both resection and structural rhinoplasty, thus leading to a new terminology, that is, preservation rhinoplasty.

PRESERVATION RHINOPLASTY FOR THE DORSUM

In order to perform a preservation technique for the nasal dorsum, the surgeon must consider the indications and contraindications (**Fig. 1**).[1]

Indications:
1. Naturally shaped dorsum with overprojection (tension nose); septum is midline
2. Short nasal bones with cartilaginous hump; normal radix position
3. Straight dorsal aesthetic lines but deviated from midline
4. Older patients with dorsal hump and thin skin envelope

Relative indications:
1. Caudal septum not in midline
2. Deformed nasal septum
3. Deep radix with a convex profile
4. Wide nasal dorsum

UNAM León, México Residence Program, León, Guanajuato, México
[1] Present address: Boulevard Campestre #703, Colonia Jardines del Moral, León, Guanajuato 37160, México.
* Corresponding author. Boulevard Campestre #703, Colonia Jardines del Moral, León, Guanajuato 37160, México.
E-mail address: contactofaces@gmail.com

Oral Maxillofacial Surg Clin N Am 33 (2021) 7–21
https://doi.org/10.1016/j.coms.2020.09.001
1042-3699/21/© 2020 Elsevier Inc. All rights reserved.

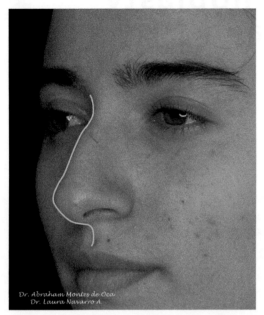

Fig. 1. Young female patient with deep radix, "S"-shaped dorsum and nasal hump. (*Courtesy of* Dr. Abraham Montes de Oca and Dr. Laura Navarro A.)

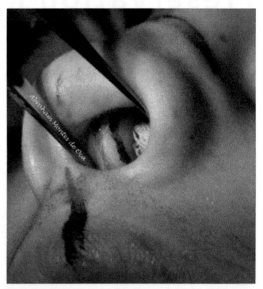

Fig. 3. The traditional or Killian incision represented by the anterior border of the septum and author technique, where the incision is made 3 to 3.5 mm posterior. (*Courtesy of* Dr. Abraham Montes de Oca.)

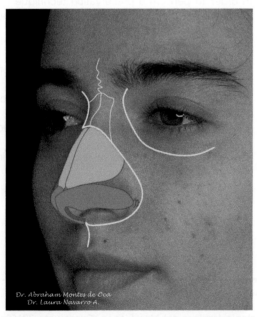

Fig. 2. Lower lateral cartilages and upper lateral cartilages differentiated by colors and its relationship with nasal and maxillary bones. (*Courtesy of* Dr. Abraham Montes de Oca and Dr. Laura Navarro A.)

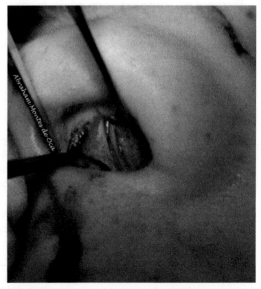

Fig. 4. The hemitransfixion incision posterior to the anterior border of the septum leaves an anterior strip of cartilage attached to the membranous septum of the anterior nasal spine of the maxillary bone. (*Courtesy of* Dr. Abraham Montes de Oca.)

5. Mildly asymmetric middle third

Contraindications:

1. Previous rhinoplasty surgery by a different surgeon
2. Previous submucous resection of the nasal septum
3. Marked third asymmetry
4. Saddle nose requiring augmentation

A decision whether to do a *push-down* (PD) procedure, whereby the osseous pyramid is squeezed and dropped inside the pyriform aperture, or a *let-down* (LD) procedure, whereby a bony segment of the nasal process of the maxilla is resected either directly or by ostectomy, depends on whether the lateral aesthetic lines need to be narrowed.[1,2] In simple words, the technique selection for the preservation rhinoplasty of the dorsum depends on the wideness. If it is adequate, the LD technique can be performed; if it is too wide, then the PD technique is indicated. The decision to use either the LD or PD technique may depend on several factors. Another consideration point for these techniques is the hump; if the dorsal hump is greater than 4 mm, then a PD technique may not be adequate for the needed descent of the nasal pyramid. Therefore, the LD

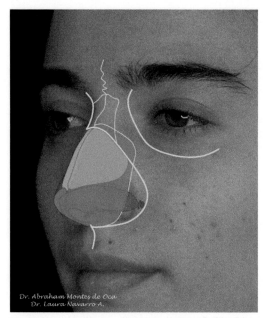

Fig. 5. Bony structures related to the nasal septum (*purple*); nasal bones, maxillary, vomer, and the perpendicular plate of ethmoid bone. (*Courtesy of* Dr. Abraham Montes de Oca and Dr. Laura Navarro A.)

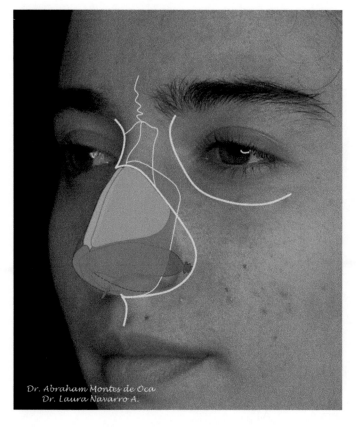

Fig. 6. The representation of the author incision for the anterior cartilage strip (posterior strut) that follows the natural shape of the septum (red arrow). (*Courtesy of* Dr. Abraham Montes de Oca and Dr. Laura Navarro A.)

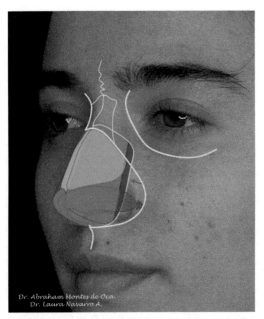

Fig. 7. The low septal strip (red) avoiding the posterior strut. (*Courtesy of* Dr. Abraham Montes de Oca and Dr. Laura Navarro A.)

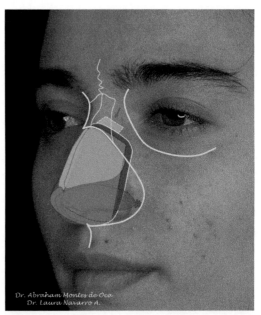

Fig. 9. All 3 resections of the cartilaginous septum (red). (1) The low septal strip, (2) posterior vertical septal strip, and a resection of the perpendicular plate of ethmoid bone below keystone area that allows a complete mobilization of the septum and a reduction of the nasal cartilaginous hump. (*Courtesy of* Dr. Abraham Montes de Oca and Dr. Laura Navarro A.)

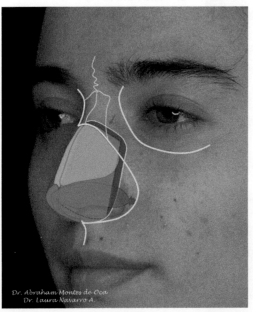

Fig. 8. The posterior septal strip (*red*). (*Courtesy of* Dr. Abraham Montes de Oca and Dr. Laura Navarro A.)

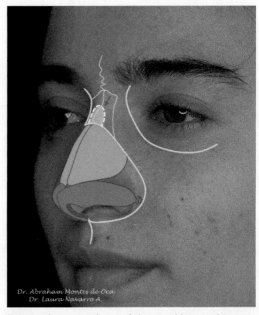

Fig. 10. The osteoplasty of the nasal bones. (*Courtesy of* Dr. Abraham Montes de Oca and Dr. Laura Navarro A.)

technique has been advocated for humps greater than 4 mm.[3]

These 2 methods of dorsal preservation can be described as follows: the PD technique basically consists of a high or low septal resection followed by lateral and transverse osteotomies, and subsequent impaction of the bony vault downward into the pyriform aperture. The LD technique consists of a high septal resection followed by resection of a portion of the ascending frontal process of the maxilla, with subsequent downward positioning of the bony vault on the process of the maxilla.

These techniques preserve the dorsum instead of the traditional structural rhinoplasty that consists of hump removal, and it can be performed under an open or close approach. If the technique is used properly, a natural nasal dorsum will be achieved, but if the techniques are overdone, then a saddle dorsum can occur.

Taking that into consideration, there are some advantages and disadvantage of dorsal preservation:

Advantages:
1. Allows both open and closed approach
2. Low septal strip allows threat of septal deviation
3. Allows a block bony pyramid rotation and mobilization

4. Preserves the anatomy of nasal dorsum and dorsal aesthetic lines
5. Natural-looking dorsum as a result, without any rhinoplasty stigma (inverted-V deformity)
6. Preserves the internal valve
7. No need for midvault reconstruction

Disadvantages:
1. Impossible to perform after the classical block hump removal
2. Septal surgery more demanding (inexperienced surgeons)

Preservation of the osseocartilaginous dorsum is in fact the biggest advance in rhinoplasty surgery (**Fig. 2**). Instead of removal of the hump by excising the dorsum, this technique lowers it by a subdorsal septal strip or caudal septal strip and by osteotomies performed over the nasal and maxillary bones.

Management of the Septum

The concept of preserving the dorsum while reducing the height of the dorsal bridge is not new. Goodale[4] reported his experience with an aesthetic case of dorsal reduction that preserved the dorsum using a combination of a high septal strip excision and PD technique, and 2 years later, he followed up this case report with a series of 22 posttraumatic rhinoplasties using a similar "push-over" technique.[4,5] Then, over the next century,

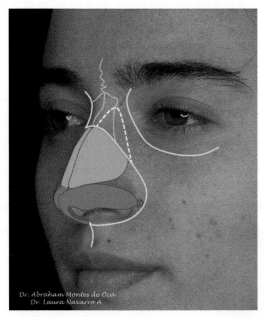

Fig. 11. Paramedian and lateral osteotomies for a reduction of the dorsal width without disarticulation of the upper lateral cartilages. (*Courtesy of* Dr. Abraham Montes de Oca and Dr. Laura Navarro A.)

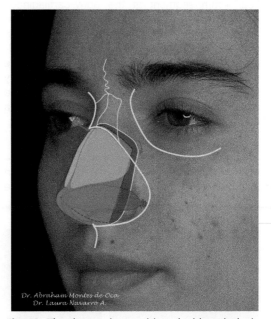

Fig. 12. The dorsum is repositioned with a clockwise rotation in order to lower the dorsal hump and improve nasal tip projection. (*Courtesy of* Dr. Abraham Montes de Oca and Dr. Laura Navarro A.)

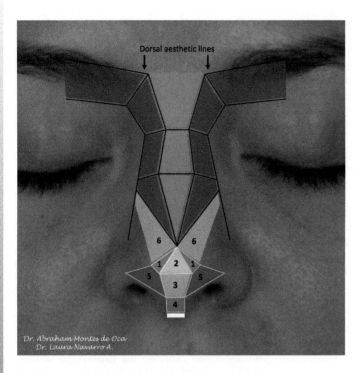

Dorsal aesthetic lines

Dr. Abraham Montes de Oca
Dr. Laura Navarro A.

Fig. 13. Nose tip polygons. (1) Dome triangle, (2) interdomal triangle, (3) infralobular polygon, (4) columellar polygon, (5) facet polygon, (6) lateral crus polygon. (*Courtesy of* Dr. Abraham Montes de Oca and Dr. Laura Navarro A.)

the concept of PD technique was used by Cottle. The Cottle PD technique favored a tripartite septal excision.[6]

An alternative to subdorsal cartilage resection classically consisted of a 3-part resection: (1) vertical 4-mm segment at the bony-cartilaginous junction (from keystone to vomer), (2) triangular resection of the ethmoid bone, and (3) inferior strip of cartilage along the maxillary spine (corresponding to the amount of desired dorsal reduction). The remaining nasal septum is sutured to the maxillary spine. This technique is the technique used by the authors in terms of preference to perform a dorsum preservation rhinoplasty.

Exposure

In the traditional technique, the hemitransfixion incision or Killian incision was performed in the anterior border of the septum; in the authors' technique, the incision takes place 3 to 3.5 mm posterior involving the total thickness of the septum and leaving the anterior portion fixed and attached to the membranous septum; then, mucoperichondrial tunnels are performed on both sides of the septum involving the cartilage portion, vomer, and ethmoidal perpendicular plate; also, inferior tunnels must involve the maxillary crest (**Figs. 3 and 4**).

Septal Cartilage Resection

After exposure of the septal cartilage is achieved, resection can be performed. A low septal strip in a wedge fashion is completed by a transversal incision in the basal portion of the septal cartilage, taking special attention around the projection of this resection in the final result of the aesthetic

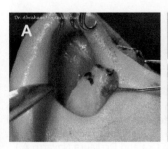
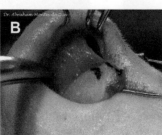

Fig. 14. The preservation of Pitanguy ligament after subperichondrial dissection of lower lateral cartilages. (*Courtesy of* Dr. Abraham Montes de Oca.)

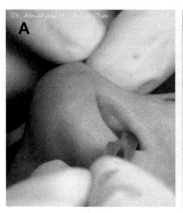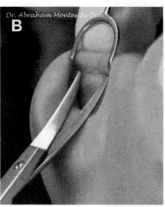

Fig. 15. The authors' technique: marginal incision (*A*) and dissection (*B*).

dorsum and its hump reduction. Taking this into consideration, the strip must be wider at the bony-cartilaginous junction; then, the strip is disarticulated from the maxillary bone (**Figs. 5–7**).

When the low septal strip is completed, the cartilaginous septum is disarticulated from the perpendicular plate of ethmoid at the bony-cartilaginous junction (from keystone area to vomer), and then a vertical posterior incision is made to remove 3 mm of the posterior cartilaginous septum in order to take a septal strip.

In that way, the septum is turned into a cartilaginous flap that remains attached to the upper later cartilages but free in the anterior posterior and lower border, which allows the septum to be moved to any desired position (**Fig. 8**). Also, a resection of the ethmoid bone below the keystone area can be performed to allow the PD/LD movement (**Fig. 9**).

In the authors' technique, the disarticulation of the upper lateral cartilages from the pyriform aperture is avoided. The authors' preference is to mobilize the bone and cartilages en bloc. That is achieved with the paramedial and lateral osteotomies.

Bony Pyramid Reduction and Movilization

The "S"-shaped dorsum denotes a challenge at this step of the surgery. To achieve better results, it is the authors' predilection to complete an osteoplasty of the bony hump at the rhinion area to adapt it to a "V"-shaped dorsum. Then, if the bony dorsum is too wide, a series of osteotomies are performed. Then, paramedian osteotomies

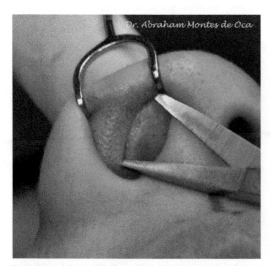

Fig. 16. Incision and dissection for lower lateral cartilages. (*Courtesy of* Dr. Abraham Montes de Oca.)

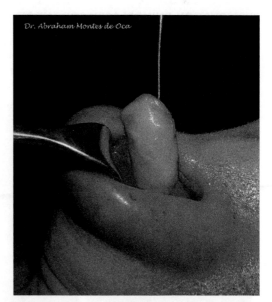

Fig. 17. Complete dissection and exposure of lower lateral cartilage by marginal approach and subperichondrial dissection. (*Courtesy of* Dr. Abraham Montes de Oca.)

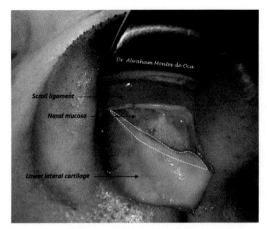

Fig. 18. Nose layers. Represented with the dashed line is the lower lateral cartilage cephalic trim. (*Courtesy of* Dr. Abraham Montes de Oca.)

(thought the dorsum) in the nasal bones followed by a lateral osteotomy (thought the pyriform aperture) in the maxillary bone are performed, allowing a bony pyramid mobilization in a PD technique that allows a transversal width reduction and improvement of dorsal aesthetic lines (**Figs. 10** and **11**).

Repositioning the Dorsum

After mobilization of the dorsum, the cartilaginous septum can be placed in any desired position to achieve movements like dorsal reduction, septal extension, septal shortening, and dorsal augmentation (**Fig. 12**).

PRESERVATION RHINOPLASTY FOR THE TIP

New developments in rhinoplasty, especially in preservation rhinoplasty, emphasize how surgeons are maintaining the soft tissues, skin,

subcutaneous layer, and the superficial musculoaponeurotic system (SMAS). The SMAS as well as its ligamentous compartments is not only a layer to be protected by careful undermining but can also be manipulated as a true flap to camouflage some cartilaginous irregularities and as a tension flap that contributes to fixating tip rotation or reducing any dead space.[7]

The aesthetically pleasing nasal tip is a composite of lines, shadows, and highlights with specific proportions and breakpoints that can be conceptualized as a series of geometric forms. Specifically, the nasal tip includes the dome triangles, the lateral crus polygons, the interdomal triangle, the facet polygons, the infralobular polygon, the columellar polygon, and the footplate polygons.[8]

The appearance of an attractive nose is created by certain lines, shadows, and highlights that cover the nasal dorsum, tip, and base. In the authors' technique, the main objective to reach these aesthetic lines and highlights, and to try to avoid the onlay grafts, if possible, is based on the Baris[8] nose tip polygons (**Fig. 13**).

Nasal Ligaments

The nasal SMAS is the third layer of the nose. Nasal vessels are running on this plane, mainly in the ligaments. The SMAS separates the nose in the superficial supra-SMAS or subskin compartment and deep sub-SMAS compartment.

The subcutaneous fat depth differs depending on the nasal areas: very thick on the radix and supratip, but thin over the K-area. This subskin layer is not the elective surgical plane for dissection.

The subperichondrical-subperiosteal dissection is bloodless and atraumatic, and the dissection is easier. In this surgical plane, it is possible to

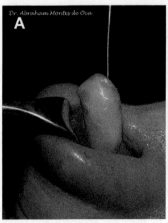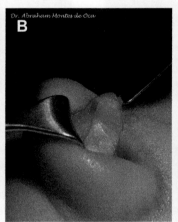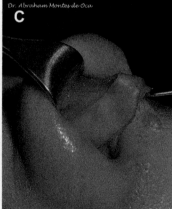

Fig. 19. (*A*) Intact lower lateral cartilage. (*B, C*) Complete cephalic and caudal trim. (*Courtesy of* Dr. Abraham Montes de Oca.)

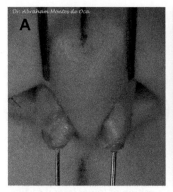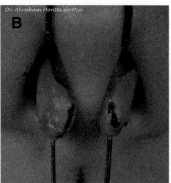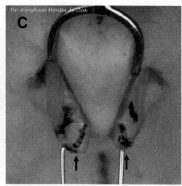

Fig. 20. (*A*) Natural aspect of domes after subperichondrial dissection. (*B*) Natural domes. (*C*) New position of the domes (*arrow*) stealing medial crus. (*Courtesy of* Dr. Abraham Montes de Oca.)

protect, repair, or reorientate the ligamentous attachments while still attached to the soft tissue.[7]

Elevation of the soft tissue envelope as a single sheet is critical to minimizing both short- and long-term problems. In addition, it is possible to preserve and/or to restore the nasal ligaments, including Pitanguy, the scroll ligament complex, and the intercrural ligament.

The nasal tip needs to be mobile. The nasal ligaments, and the Pitanguy ligament in particular, ensure elastic rotation and projection, toward the nasal tip (**Fig. 14**).

When joining the subperichondrial dissection pockets between the alar and upper lateral cartilages, it is possible to keep the scroll ligament complex intact.[5]

The preservation of the attachments of Pitanguy ligament to the underlying soft tissue at surgery has different benefits, including the improving tip

projection, shortening of the infralobular curve, and accentuating supratip break.

Surgical Approaches

In rhinoplasty, one basically needs to get access to dorsum, tip, and septum; 2 different incisions can be used, that will protect the ligaments and allow for perfect surgical exposure.

These 2 incisions allow the surgeon to bypass the Scroll ligament and the deep SMAS and leave them untouched between the alar and cephalic compartments; if requested, they can also be divided and reoriented.[7]

1. The marginal incision
   Endonasal incisions: (A) intercartilaginous, (B) intracartilaginous, (C) marginal
2. The interseptum-columnella incision, as performed in septoplasty procedures, protects the deep SMAS attachments to the anterior caudal angle and to the depressor septi nasi connections (**Figs. 15** and **16**).

Technique Description: Step by Step

Traditionally, surgeons achieved the desired tip shape using a combination of excision, incision, sutures, and grafts. Even when the results were good initially, a significant percentage of these cases deteriorated over time. The adoption of tip suturing and structural support using various columellar struts, septal extension grafts, and tongue-in-groove procedures resulted in dramatically improved intermediate-term results with maintenance of projection and fewer tip deformities. Nowadays, the preservation rhinoplasty advances tip surgery even further by preserving virtually the entire alar cartilage, which enhances function and reduces potential problems.[5]

At this point, the main purpose of preservation rhinoplasty is to maintain cartilages and ligaments

Fig. 21. Final result of lateral crural steal and transdomal sutures. Dome triangles in white. (*Courtesy of* Dr. Abraham Montes de Oca.)

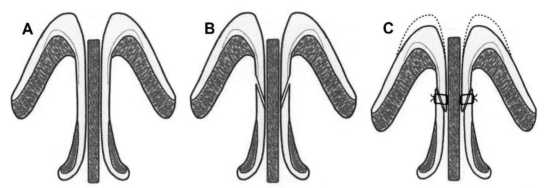

Fig. 22. The medial crus overlap to decrease the lobule projection. (*A*) Natural position of lower lateral cartilages (*blue*) and columella strut (*purple*). (*B*) Oblique incision at the columella break point. (*C*) Suture after resection or overlap technique.

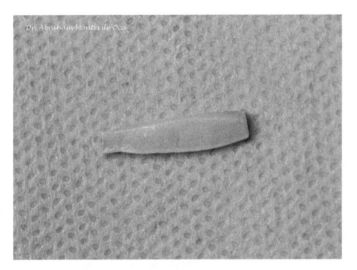

Fig. 23. Columellar strut design from septal graft. (*Courtesy of* Dr. Abraham Montes de Oca.)

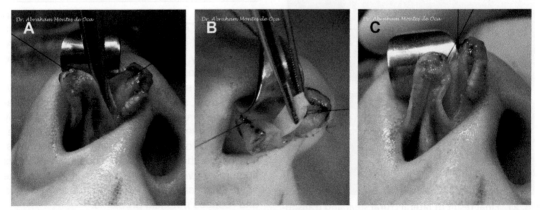

Fig. 24. Columellar strut positioning. (*A*) Pocket creation. (*B*) Placement of the columellar strut into the pocket. (*C*) Columellar strut final position. (*Courtesy of* Dr. Abraham Montes de Oca.)

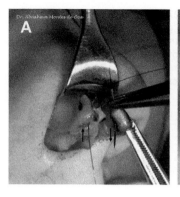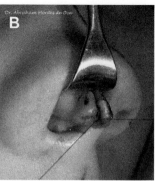

Fig. 25. Interdomal suture. (*Courtesy of Dr. Abraham Montes de Oca.*)

in order to obtain natural and stable aesthetic results.

For the preservation rhinoplasty of the tip, the authors' technique includes the next steps after the incision of the posterior septal strut is complete:

1. Exposure and dissection of lower lateral cartilages
2. Cephalic trim
3. Caudal trim
4. Transdomal suture and lateral crural steal
5. Columellar strut
6. Interdomal suture
7. Posterior strut

The subperichondrial plane of dissection in rhinoplasty is a relatively atraumatic, avascular plane that minimizes soft tissue injury, leading to decreased intraoperative edema and more predictable postoperative results.

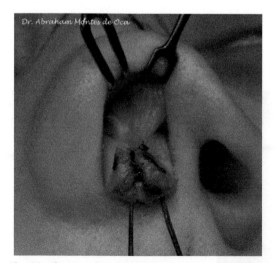

Fig. 26. The complete transdomal and interdomal suture and its effect on tip definition. (*Courtesy of* Dr. Abraham Montes de Oca.)

The exposure of lower lateral cartilages is approached by a marginal incision and a subperichondrial dissection in the aim to avoid muscles, fat, ligaments, nerves, and blood vessels located above the perichondrium within and superficial to the SMAS (**Fig. 17**).

Cephalic and Caudal Trim

Cephalic and caudal resections should be as conservative as possible, and it is important to maintain a minimum height of the inferior lateral cartilage of at least 7 mm, to reach the flattening polygon. A cephalic or caudal resection greater than 3 mm should be avoided. In the case of soft cartilages, a sliding alar cartilage flap can be done to improve their support and capability to maintain their shape after surgery (**Fig. 18**).

Cephalic and caudal trim can be performed with a 15 or 15c blade; the aim of this technique is demolding and design of the lower lateral cartilages to improve their final shape, avoiding the overresection that can lead into a pinching nose effect (**Fig. 19**).

Transdomal Suture and Lateral Crural Steal

At this point, the Pitanguy ligament remains attached to the SMAS at the supratip breaking point. After the lower lateral cartilages design by the cephalic and caudal trim is complete, the transdomal suture takes place to project the nasal tip by equalization and repositioning of the domes.

To project, define, and reshape the nasal tip, a transdomal suture can be done.

The most common technique to achieve projection is the lateral crural steal, whereby the domes are repositioned medially into the medial crus to gain height, and new domes are created stealing lateral crus, into a medial position. The new position of the domes is fixed with a nylon 5-0 cephalic dome suture (**Figs. 20** and **21**).

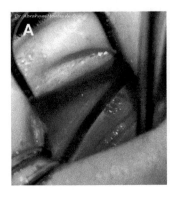
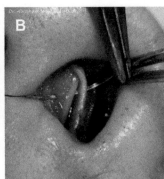

Fig. 27. Posterior strut. (*A*) The incision and gap between the cartilaginous septum and the posterior strut. (*B*) Suture of the posterior strut into desire position. (*Courtesy of* Dr. Abraham Montes de Oca.)

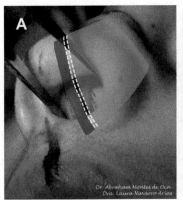
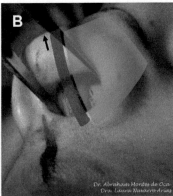
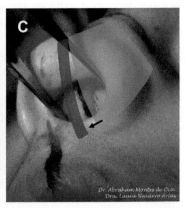

Fig. 28. (*A*) Posterior strut and cartilaginous septum after incision. The posterior strut can be fixed to anterior septal angle in an upper or lower position (*B*) or can be rotated in a longitudinal plane (*C*) to modify the final tip projection. (*Courtesy of* Dr. Abraham Montes de Oca and Dr. Laura Navarro A.)

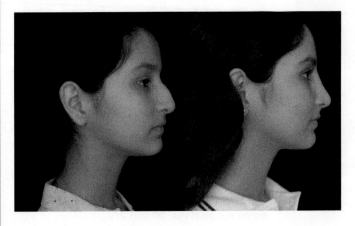

Fig. 29. A case of preservation rhinoplasty. Young female patient with an "S sapped" dorsum, profile view. Preoperative and postoperative.

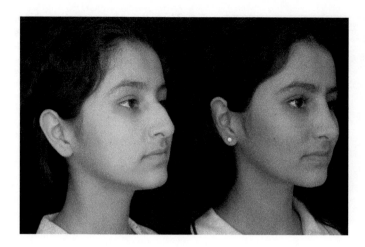

Fig. 30. A case of preservation rhinoplasty. Young female patient with an "S sapped" dorsum, three-quarter view. Preoperative and postoperative.

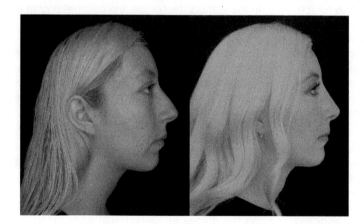

Fig. 31. A case of preservation rhinoplasty. Profile view. Preoperative and postoperative.

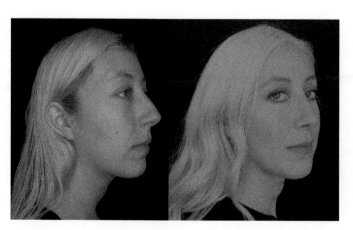

Fig. 32. A case of preservation rhinoplasty. Three-quarter view. Preoperative and postoperative.

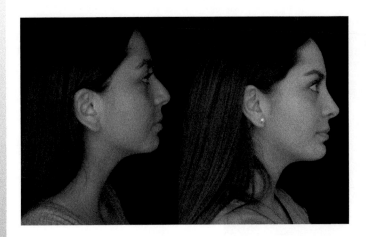

Fig. 33. A case of preservation rhinoplasty with very natural results, profile view. Preoperative and postoperative.

In cases of overprojected noses, the most efficient treatment of long lobule is a medial crural overlap, and the most convenient location for it is the columella break point.[7] An oblique incision from caudal to posterior at the columella break point increases the cut contact surface. Dissect the cut cartilage ends for 2 to 3 mm from the mucosa to achieve overlap, and then the medial crus is tucked under the middle crus to obtain an overlap of 2 to 3 mm and is fixed with a 5-0 nylon suture (**Fig. 22**).

Columellar Strut

A common reason for loss of rotation is an inadequate tip support. The reason is that the columellar strut is the elective technique to improve support, rotation, and projection of the nasal tip, avoiding the lateral crus excision and the onlay grafts.

The complete technique has its origin in the pioneering work of Regalado-Briz an Byrd.[9] Regalado-Briz describes it as a tip suturing technique with a columellar strut that results in a symmetric unified supported tip complex.

In the authors' technique, the columellar graft is sculpted from the low septal strip previously performed in the dorsal preservation rhinoplasty.

The columella must have a balanced position in relation to the adjacent alar rim and medial crura. In addition to the aesthetic, the columella provides a central scaffold on which the adjacent structures retain support and balance (**Figs. 23** and **24**).[10]

Interdomal Suture

The interdomal suture provides tip strength and symmetry. This stitch is particularly important if the domes are weak and tend to splay apart; however, the purpose of the interdomal suture is not to bring the domes in contact with each other. An interdomal suture brings the tips together, prevents them from splaying, and contributes to the narrowing of the nasal tip. The purchase is made posterior to the domes. Usually the cephalic

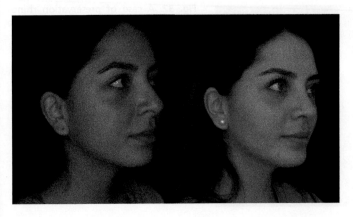

Fig. 34. A case of preservation rhinoplasty showing the dorsal line improvement with natural results, three-quarter view. Preoperative and postoperative.

ends of the domes can be separated from one another by about 3 mm.[1]

The overall nasal tip width is controlled by the interdomal suture as well as the transdomal sutures.

The authors' preference for the interdomal suture is performed with a 5-0 nylon (**Figs. 25 and 26**).

Posterior Strut

At the end of the surgery, the posterior strut, which was separated from the cartilaginous septum in the dorsal preservation surgery, is fixed in the desired position according to the individual requirements. If more rotation is needed, the posterior strut slides over the cartilaginous septum to a cephalic position and is fixed to the anterior septal angle, with a 4-0 nylon suture. If the objective is to reduce tip projection, the opposite maneuver is performed (toward caudal) (**Figs. 27** and **28**).

Once the posterior strut is fixed, the authors' preference is to perform a transeptal suture instead of nasal packing in order to avoid bleeding or septal hematoma, reduce edema, close the dead space, and provide internal support.

The preservation rhinoplasty is considered an innovative technique with exponential growth among nose surgeons worldwide. This technique can provide every patient with very stable and satisfactory results and avoids the stigma of an operated nose. The preservation of structures, such as cartilages, ligaments, and the osseocartilaginous dorsum, lead the surgeon into very natural aesthetic lines and nasal polygons, but to achieve these results and the adequate management of the technique, the surgeon must have an extensive knowledge of surgical anatomy, must have special surgical abilities, and must be capable of developing several techniques (**Figs. 29–34**).

DISCLOSURE

The authors have nothing to disclose.

REFERENCES

1. Saban Y, Daniel RK, Polselli R, et al. Dorsal preservation: the push down technique reassessed. Aesthet Surg J 2018;38:117–31.
2. Rollin DK. Preservation Rhinoplasty: Rational & Overview. In: Saban Y, Çakir B, Daniel R, et al, editors. Preservation Rhinoplasty. Bio Ofset. 2018;18-29.
3. Tuncel U, Aydogdu O. The probable reasons for dorsal hump problems following let-down/push-down rhinoplasty and solution proposals. Plast Reconstr Surg 2019;144(3):378e–85e.
4. Goodale JL. The correction of old lateral displacements of the nasal bones. Boston Medical and Surgical Journal 1901;20:538–9.
5. Daniel R, Kosins A. Current trends in preservation rhinoplasty. Aesthetic Surgery Journal Open Forum 2020.
6. Cottle MH. Nasal roof repair and hump removal. AMA Arch Otolaryngol 1954;60(4):408–14.
7. B Cakir, Y Saban, R Daniel, et al. Preservation rhinoplasty. 2018; 163–212.
8. Cakır B, Öreroğlu AR, Rollin DR. Surface aesthetics in tip rhinoplasty: a step-by-step guide. Aesthet Surg J 2014;34:941–55.
9. Regalado-Briz A, Byrd SH. Aesthetic rhinoplasty with maximum preservation of alar cartilages: experience with 52 consecutive cases. Plast Reconstr Surg 1999;103(2):671–80 [discussion: 681–2].
10. Rohrich RJ, Hoxworth RE, Kurkjian TJ. The role of the columellar strut in rhinoplasty. Plast Reconstr Surg 2012;129(1):118e–25e.

Piezoelectric Technology in Rhinoplasty

Seied Omid Keyhan, DDS, OMFS[a],*, Behnaz Poorian, DDS, OMFS[b,1],
Hamid Reza Fallahi, DDS, OMFS[c,d,2]

KEYWORDS

- Piezosurgery • Osteotomy • Rhinoplasty • Septoplasty

KEY POINTS

- In piezosurgery, a frequency of 25 to 29 kHz cuts only mineralized tissue and frequencies greater than 50 kHz cut neurovascular tissue and other soft tissues.
- The philosophy of applying the ultrasonic surgical devices in rhinoplasty decreases postsurgical sequelae (ecchymosis, edema, pain).
- Complete degloving of the nasal bone is not necessary for piezoelectric rhinoplasty.
- Endonasal or external lateral osteotomy could be performed with piezosurgery.
- Cost and learning curves are the main disadvantages of piezosurgery.

INTRODUCTION

The title of ultrasound determines the mechanical vibrations in frequencies higher than the human upper audible limit, which is higher than 20 Khz. Piezosurgery is based on the piezoelectric effect, in which an electric polarization is generated against mechanical stress in certain crystals and ceramics.

Piezoelectric tools have been used in bone surgeries since the last 20 years. It is appropriate for all bony surgery; however, it is most beneficial for the restricted access and/or the bones adjacent to the delicate soft tissues (nerves, vessels, mucosa, skin, pleura, and dura). Initially, piezoelectric was used in oral and dental surgical processes such as third molar extraction, excision of cysts, the formation of an opening into the maxillary sinus, preparing implant sites, and lifting the periosteum. Consequently, piezoelectric was used in maxillofacial surgery with extension to mandibular sagittal split osteotomies, temporomandibular joint surgery, cranial bone harvesting, and maxillary LeFort I osteotomies. Piezoelectric is chiefly effective in craniofacial surgery, as it permits the surgeon to do extensive osteotomies without damage to the adjacent neurovascular structures and underlying dura. Accordingly, applications of the standard use of piezoelectric in many different fields of surgery such as otological surgery (chain replacement and stapedectomy and facial nerve decompression), orthopedic surgery (osteotomy and hardware removal), and rhinoplasty have been launched. Various piezoelectric working tips have been laid out for currently available indications.[1,2]

FUNDAMENTAL SCIENCE

Ultrasonic transduction is the principle of ultrasonic bone cutting, which is afforded by piezoelectric ceramic contraction and expansion, and

[a] Cranio-Maxillo-Facial Research Center for Craniofacial Reconstruction, Tehran University of Medical Sciences, Shariati Hospital, Tehran, Iran; [b] Private Practice; [c] Dental Research Center, Research Institute of Dental Sciences, Shahid Beheshti University of Medical Science, Tehran, Iran; [d] School of Advanced Technologies in Medicine, Shahid Beheshti University of Medical Sciences
[1] present address: Unit 403, #7, Varasteh Avn, next to the Hojjat Soori Alley, Darrous, Teharn 1949843313, Iran.
[2] present address: 3rd floor, Jame-Jam medical tower, east pahlevan, kianpars ST, Ahvaz 986155683651, Iran
* Corresponding author. Unit 3, floor1, Mahtab building, Mahtab Alley, shahid ebrahimzadeh Alley(#11), west hasht behesht ST, Bozormehr ST, Isfahan 8154748915, Iran
E-mail address: keyhanomid@ymail.com

Oral Maxillofacial Surg Clin N Am 33 (2021) 23–30
https://doi.org/10.1016/j.coms.2020.09.002
1042-3699/21/© 2020 Elsevier Inc. All rights reserved.

making microvibrations. Essentially, they are modified by the transmission of an electric current across given crystals and ceramics leading to the oscillations that are then amplified and conveyed to a vibrating insert. Through suction irrigation, bony tissue is emulsified and eliminated without mechanical or thermal damage to the adjacent tissue. Adjusting the ultrasonic frequency at a low level causes the metallic insert for oscillating the cutting hard tissues (cartilages, bones) while leaving remaining soft tissues untouched (nerves, vessels, mucous membranes). The insert's tip shakes within a range of 60 to 200 μm, permitting a very accurate bone incision. A frequency of 25 to 29 kHz is used, as only mineralized tissue is cut by the micromovements formed at this frequency; neurovascular tissue and other soft tissues are cut at frequencies greater than 50 kHz.

Piezoelectric tools normally include the main power unit and a foot switch and handpiece that are linked to it. This includes a holder for the handpiece containing irrigation fluids creating a modifiable jet of 0 to 60 mL/min through a peristaltic pump. It eliminates debris from the cutting area and guarantees accurate cutting. It also keeps a blood-free operation area as a result of cavitation of the irrigation solution and provides better visibility mainly in complex anatomic areas. The cutting features of the piezosurgery tool need to be set in terms of the level of bone mineralization, the design of the used insert, the speed of movement over usage, and the pressure used on the handpiece.[2,3]

TISSUES' BIOLOGICAL REACTION

A piezoelectric tool contains numerous advantages for preparing the periosteum, based on the reports of some studies. Subperiosteal preparation and bone cutting by the piezoelectric device is associated with a positive influence on bone metabolism, faster healing, and bone regeneration, in comparison to the results of the conventional periosteal elevator, diamond, or carbide drills. Oxygen molecules sent out over cutting have an ultrasonic vibration and antiseptic impact and stimulate cellular metabolism. By the precision in the osteotomy, it is allowed to preserve the normal bone architecture, a factor contributing to the acceleration of bone regeneration. This positive effect of piezoelectric on bone remodeling in patients with comorbidities or treated with chemotherapeutic agents, bisphosphonates, or other medications should be investigated.[4–6]

Some investigators have also pointed out that bone extracted from osteotomies conducted with a piezo device included more osteocytes and more vital bone than bone attained with usual methods.[7]

The perfusion in osseous vessels in the bloodless piezoelectric bone cutting field was investigated by Von See and colleagues. Local overheating, cavitation effects, the flow of the cooling fluid, or intravascular thrombosis caused by the use of piezoelectric tools were assumed as the possible justification for the bloodless osteotomy site. Damage to vascular cell walls and standing waves in the vessels following the use of ultrasound and platelets aggregation (thrombus organization) are other assumptions that could reduce or even cutoff microvascular perfusion completely and lead to local infarction with subsequent necrosis. As a result of these investigations, the cavitation effects that are the formation of sound-induced gas bubbles and cavities at the negative peak pressure of an ultrasonic wave would be the main reason for the relative absence of blood, and the other probable aforementioned mechanisms are unlikely to occur at ultrasonic osteotomy site.[6] Furthermore, it was histologically shown that bony surfaces cut with piezoelectric are present by a lack of coagulation necrosis by preserving osteocytes. This property proves the potential of piezoelectric in performing osteotomy, maintaining the low risk of osteonecrosis as a result of the selective and micrometric cutting action.[8]

PIEZOELECTRIC RHINOPLASTY

The philosophy of applying the ultrasonic surgical devices in rhinoplasty decreases the postsurgical sequence (ecchymosis, edema, pain), maximizes the precision, and increases overall patient comfort. Patient satisfaction is imperative in aesthetic processes, and the surgeon's motivation to use new approaches is enhanced by patient satisfaction.

Osteotomy is one of the most procedure-sensitive phases in rhinoplasty surgery and sturdily influences the patient's clinical outcome, based on not only surgical results but also the safety and lack of complications. As established in the literature, edema and ecchymosis are straightly relative to the degree of soft tissue injury and the mechanical trauma to the bony surface over the osteotomies and skeletonizing. Surgeons for diminishing these inconveniences sequel have examined various methods, instruments, and intra- and postoperative materials and methods.[2,9–11]

In conventional rhinoplasty surgery, management of the lateral walls and the bony vault is mostly conducted by mechanical tools including saws, osteotomes, chisels, and rasps that are independent of their design and greatly vulnerable to distracting major blood vessels in the soft tissues surrounding the nasal bone. These tools were refined for minimizing damage to the adjacent soft tissues and maximizing accuracy, over the years. Nevertheless, a search for more accurate surgical tools was prompted by the sustained absence of accuracy and the related uncontrollable fracture lines. Afterward, for overcoming the restrictions of manual instruments, electric tools with reciprocating heads were established. Surgeons use a piezoelectric technique for the management of different steps of rhinoplasty such as the lateral and bony vault osteotomy, deepening of the radix/glabellar, anterior nasal spine resection, correction of bony asymmetries, septoplasty, and turbinoplasty.[5,9,12,13]

The initial cadaver study reported on using a piezo scalpel in rhinoplasty was published by Robiony in 2007, who performed lateral osteotomies via a percutaneous method (**Fig. 1**), and the advantages including a minimal periosteal detachment, minimal or lacking internal mucosal damage, and the rapid linear cut were considered. Followed by their previous study, further study was conducted by investigators for more investigation on this issue. Their studies indicated that

piezosurgery is a simply managed tool, along with the significant decrease in postoperative edema, trauma, and ecchymosis confirming the strict association between minor surgical trauma and better hard and soft tissue performance over healing.[10]

Another human cadaveric experiment was performed by Ghassemi and colleagues. They used the special tool tip as a periosteal elevator for creating a subperiosteal tunnel around the pyriform aperture along the planned osteotomy track. The piezo scalpel was put within this tunnel, and the osteotomy was carried out alongside the osteotomy path with digital control. They mentioned that the piezosurgical scalpel is highly effective, easy to handle, controllable, and nontraumatic substitute for known osteotomy methods and does not lead to any mucosa laceration. The osteotomy with piezotome is carried out accurately in the intended osteotomy track, not resulting in any comminuted properties. Although requiring probably a learning curve, it is a straightforward technique to learn.[12]

Only a few reports exist on controlled investigations that compare the piezoelectric nasal bone cut with the traditional method. Tirelli and colleagues compared the conventional osteotome and piezosurgery in 22 candidates undergoing rhinoplasty through an external method for osteotomy. The surgeon conducted a 2-mm long incision 8 to 10 mm below and medially to the medial canthus, including the skin, the periosteum, and the underlying superficial muscular aponeurotic system tissues. A narrow, curved, and unguarded tip of the piezoelectric was put via the pilot incision up to the nasal bone. Before activating, the tip was manually pushed caudally and cranially into the incision to create minimal periosteal detachment, limited to the considered line of the lateral osteotomy without requiring a subperiosteal tunnel. Edema and ecchymosis existed in the primary postoperative periods, only in 2 patients (20%) from the piezosurgery group in comparison to 12 patients (83%) from the usual technique group. This is another evidence that has mentioned a lower rate of postoperative morbidities with the piezosurgery application.

This study showed the osteotomies conducted with the piezoelectric seemed to be further linear, accurate, and efficient compared with those carried out with the traditional osteotome, particularly in the subjects with a wide nasal dorsum and thicker nasal bones.[8]

Koc and colleagues represented the outcomes of a trial comparing the clinical outcomes of the ultrasonic external osteotomies with usual internal osteotomies. The 2 groups were compared based

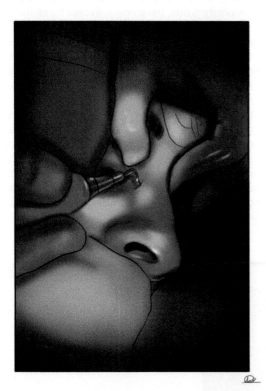

Fig. 1. Percutaneous lateral wall osteotomy by piezosurgery.

on the duration of surgery, postoperative edema, perioperative bleeding, pain, ecchymosis, and patient satisfaction on the first and seventh postoperative days. The piezosurgery group indicated considerably more favorable outcomes based on edema, hemorrhage, and ecchymosis on the first day postoperatively. On the contrary, ecchymosis and edema were also better on the seventh postoperative day in the piezosurgery group. Hemorrhage was the same in both groups on the seventh postoperative day. In the piezosurgery group, not only less pain was experienced on the first postoperative day, but also these patients were more pleased with their outcomes on both the first and seventh postoperative days. Based on the results of the current work, it is implied that piezosurgery is probably a safe, promising, and effective technique for lateral osteotomy, a critical stage in rhinoplasty. The satisfaction and comfort of both surgeons and patients counteract the time interval essential for the learning curve.[14]

Taskın and colleagues assessed postoperative ecchymosis and edema in their double-blinded prospective work in patients undergoing open rhinoplasty and endonasal lateral wall osteotomy with piezoelectric as opposed usual tools. The whole subperiosteal degloving of the whole nasal bone was performed up to the medial canthus, nasion, and nasal maxillary sulcus in all patients, not related to the kind of used osteotomy tool (**Fig. 2**). On the second day, the edema scores were considerably incremented in comparison to the seventh day in both groups. Nevertheless, no considerable difference was found between groups. In postoperative day 2, the ecchymosis scores were slightly higher in comparison to that on day 7; in both groups, however, it was not significant statistically. In this work, it was indicated that the main reason for ecchymosis and edema observed after rhinoplasty is associated with the soft tissue injury. This is clarified by the whole subperiosteal degloving of the complete nasal bone leading to extreme soft tissue manipulation, essentially boosting the risk of edema irrespective

of the conduction of the osteotomies with the traditional or ultrasonic method. However, despite the complete degloving of nasal bone by preventing soft tissue injury over osteotomy and diminishing the severity of ecchymosis, regardless of the used osteotomy tools, it should be expected to extend the recovery from edema. Other comparable investigations are required to assess the effectiveness of complete degloving of nasal bone in avoiding ecchymosis and edema.[9] On the other hand, Fallahi and colleagues executed the double-blinded, randomized controlled trial for comparing the postoperative pain, ecchymosis, and edema in internal lateral osteotomies conducted using the piezosurgery tool with that using conventional technique. Surgeries started as a regular open rhinoplasty to perform a lateral osteotomy, submucosal tunnel with no complete nasal bone degloving made along the nasal surface of the maxilla's ascending process in the same mode for both groups (**Fig. 3**). Based on the results, doing internal lateral osteotomy via the piezosurgery tool is accompanied by the lower postoperative pain, ecchymosis, and edema in comparison to the usual osteotomy.[15]

Troedhan and colleagues also designated the other prospective comparative investigation between piezotome rhinoplasty and rhinoplasty with traditional tools and protocols. In the piezotome rhinoplasty group, the surgery, except for skin incisions, was carried out only with different surgical ultrasonic tips. Through the cavitation impact of ultrasonic surgical tools, the periosteal detachment from nasal bone with ultrasonic periosteal elevators and the atraumatic supraperichondrial dissection of nasal dermal soft tissues with blunt ultrasonic tips are mainly enabled. The exact and undisruptive separation of periosteum and tissue layers was performed by the rhythmic microscopic oscillating pressure waves. This work includes the results comparable to the other studies and points out the highest soft tissue preservation, lack of complications such as bruising and bleeding, and exact modeling of the nasal bone with

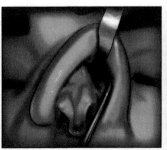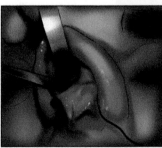

Fig. 2. Endonasal piezoelectric lateral wall osteotomy by complete degloving of nasal bone.

from navigation-directed rhinoplasty. On the contrary, preoperative computed tomographic scan is improbable for rhinoplasty candidate with esthetic aims; hence, they would not be appropriate for the navigational method. More comparative studies are required to investigate the outcome differences between the piezoelectric and piezonavigated methods.[11]

ULTRASONIC RHINOSCULPTURE

Some investigators explained using the piezoelectric tool for the 3-dimensional bone reshaping of the nasal dorsum (particularly when the bony vault needed only a slight decrease [1–3 mm]) and by incremental bony refinements without damaging adjacent structures with related narrowing to meet superior visualization for obtaining excellent cosmetic and functional outcomes. Sonic rhinoplasty under direct visualization allows for a precise, safe, low-impact sculpting of the nasal bones with an exclusive ability for shaping the mobile bony segment after osteotomy.[1,2,17]

DISCUSSION AND CONCLUSION

Piezoelectric tools are the novel ultrasonic methods for effective and safe osteoplasty or osteotomy in comparison with traditional soft and hard tissue approaches using rotating instruments due to lack of microvibrations, ease of control and use, and safer cutting, mainly in complex anatomic areas. Numerous clinical advantages are obtained by its mechanical and physical features, including precise cutting, better visualization of the surgical field, and sparing the vital neurovascular bundles. Piezoelectric bone surgery seems to be more effective in the first steps of bony healing, by providing an earlier bone morphogenetic proteins uptake, stimulates remodeling of bone, and controls the inflammatory procedure as well.

Adopting novel methods in rhinoplasty surgery can be complex or simple.[12] The piezoelectric device is an innovative surgical instrument using piezoelectric ultrasonic vibrations to cut the tissues with a high level of accuracy from the 2 past decades. It was used in both closed and open rhinoplasty procedures. The piezoelectric device could be used in different steps in rhinoplasty surgery from the dissection with various especial design tips to turbinoplasty, cap removal, radix reduction, nasal spine manipulation, and lateral osteotomy. Anatomically, the dorsal hump incorporates a cartilaginous vault that has been covered with a bony cap. Frequently, the bony hump removal with an osteotome could result in

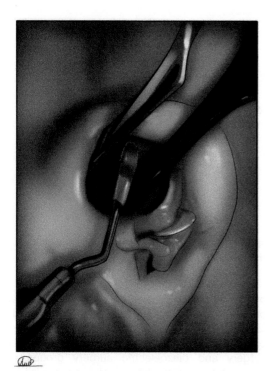

Fig. 3. Endonasal piezoelectric lateral wall osteotomy by creating subperiosteal tunnel around the pyriform aperture along the planned osteotomy track.

ultrasonic surgical tools and the greater cosmetic as a result of smoothness and symmetry of the nasal dorsum.[16]

In 2019, Robiony proposed the piezonavigated method, as a development of their original piezosurgical external method. In this technique, the straight view of the operation field and complementary positional guidance, not practicable with the traditional external method, could be provided by navigation system. The use of this technology to the operating setting could result in the further benefits of the original piezosurgical method, not by altering the surgical method but also by facilitating the surgeon to do the desired osteotomy line. Furthermore, using this technology in rhinoplasty would not provide an economic burden, because navigation systems are used by numerous craniofacial surgery and ear, throat, and nose units presently for trauma, reconstructive, oncologic, and endoscopic surgery. Nevertheless, such a method should be regarded only for greatly complex cases requiring preoperative imaging even not performing navigation. Particularly, such a method could be beneficial for facial malformation and posttraumatic nasal deformity needing cautious preoperative surgical planning. Moreover, patients with obstructive symptoms who need functional procedures could profit the injury to the underlying cartilaginous vault or an "open roof" prolonging 6 to 10 mm cephalic to the keystone junction. Conversely, gradual bony cap reduction is performed by the piezosurgery without damaging the underlying cartilage or creating an open roof. In this case, if the spreader flaps used, it can be extended cephalically in the bony vault, leading to a more natural dorsal reconstruction. Similarly, any sharp spicules or edges followed by osteotomies can be simply removed using piezoelectric even on mobilized bones. Generally, removal of lateral edge of bony cap with optional extension onto the lateral sidewall is done by piezoelectric, for which the considerable consequence is afforded as a result of this extension: (1) it permits the cephalic dorsal lines followed by hump decrease defined by cartilage instead of the bony lateral wall, and (2) it makes it possible to shape the cephalic cartilaginous vault with sutures, thus reducing the requirement for medial oblique osteotomies to adapt and narrow the dorsal bony vault. Lateral osteotomy could be performed whether existing internal or external with or without subperiosteal tunneling along the osteotomy line with a piezoelectric device. By piezotechnology, the need to aid the surgeon in conducting osteotomies, therefore, both assistant and force variations from mallet strikes will be omitted.[2]

The piezosurgery has the ability to exactly choose the target tissue, make it possible the optimal detachment of the periosteum and separation of the soft tissue layers. Consequently, the histologic base of the periosteum remains intact preserving its function as well as the risk of disrupting delicate structures such as blood vessels, mucosal membranes, and nerves are maintained at a minimum. Therefore, ecchymosis, bleeding, and edema become negligible. Histologically, it was indicated that the piezotome does not result in bone coagulation necrosis and maintains the osteocyte microscopically intact. Furthermore, the piezotome contributes to improving the postsurgical microcirculation in comparison to the traditional periosteal elevators. Some investigators have indicated that the main reason for ecchymosis over osteotomy is damage to the angular artery or vein at the level of the medial canthus. Based on this theory, impending such delicate structures through more precise instruments, such as the piezotome over piezosurgery, would considerably lead to the lower periorbital ecchymosis[7,18](**Fig. 4**).

Few studies indicated no considerable difference between the 2 methods based on objective outcomes. Taskın and colleagues in their study performed the complete subperiosteal degloving

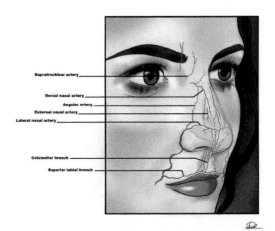

Fig. 4. Nasal vessels may be damaged during rhinoplasty.

of the whole nasal bone and endonasal lateral osteotomy with piezoelectric under direct visualization. However, in this work, no related difference was found between the conventional surgery and piezoelectric surgery groups. It could be clarified by the comprehensive subperiosteal degloving of the whole nasal bone. Although the whole degloving of nasal bone by preventing soft tissue injury over osteotomy may reduce the ecchymosis severity, the excessive elevation of periosteum intrinsically tends to increment the risk of edema, without considering the conduction of the osteotomies with the traditional or ultrasonic method. Gerbault and colleagues advocate the extensive exposure of nasal bone during performing rhinoplasty with a piezoelectric device. They believe that more precise analysis and surgical correction of disfigurements of the osseocartilaginous vault could be performed by the wide exposure. Moreover, they reported another benefit of performing wide exposure, as (1) lateral bony wall asymmetry is straightly managed by piezosurgery instead of only by breaking the bone, (2) all kinds of osteotomies are carried out more exactly without risk of radiating fracture lines, which happens with chisels and osteotomes, (3) osteotomies and rasping are conducted on thin or brittle bones and on mobilized lateral bony walls with no risk of disruption, (4) the complete osteotomies are carried out with stability, as the underlying mucosa and periosteum are not damaged, and it is difficult to avoid this damage with conventional methods.[2] Contrarily, from the Robiony's studies perspective, an adequate guaranty of nasal bone vascularization is not provided by such a method, in terms of wide stripping of the periosteum from the nasal bone, and it could lead to the reduced bone healing, with resultant step deformities as the everlasting documents of bone resorption, probably decreasing the benefits conveyed by using piezosurgery.[10,11,19]

Piezosurgery includes the main disadvantages as the high cost, prolonged operating time, and learning curve.[7,18] Originally, the increased operation time is probably 30 minutes as a result of the required elevation of the soft tissue envelope and controlled visualizing the osteotomies. Based on the experience, the surgeon can implement these steps faster and the accuracy of the surgical steps conducted with the piezoelectric results in fewer correction later in the operating sequence. Similar to the adoption of any new method, modifications exist in the operative method and a learning curve for instrumenting. Studies indicate that the piezosurgery is straightforward to learn and increasing the learning curves of the practicing surgeons will result in the less significant difference in the length of surgery between the 2 methods. Furthermore, as a result of the Robiony's 10-year piezoelectric rhinoplasty experiments, this slight increase in the length of surgery would be entirely balanced by the benefits in surgical accuracy and postoperative sequelae indicated by this method.[11]

SUMMARY

According to the results of the many studies and the investigators' experiences, it could be indicated that the piezosurgery in rhinoplasty can be considered as a reliable and safe method and should be taken into account as a part of the surgeon's repertoire for rhinoplasty. Piezoelectric, a recent instrument in an osteotomy, indicates favorable and valuable outcomes based on the immediate postoperative morbidities, even though, long-term results have not been investigated. Nevertheless, further randomized controlled trials are required to explain the piezosurgery relative merits against usual osteotomy considering the long-term aesthetic results and patient satisfaction. Recently, the possibility of using a combination of piezosurgery and navigation to adjust the osteotomy line position, mostly in a subgroup of complex cases, has been suggested by Robiony and his colleagues due to their cadaver and clinical experience during 10 years.

CLINICS CARE POINTS

- During piezoelectric surgery, proper irrigation system is mandatory.

- During piezoelectric surgery, avoiding from excess pressure on working head should be considered.
- During piezoelectric surgery, one should be patient.
- This is an auxiliary technology not a revelation and necessity.

DISCLOSURE

The authors have nothing to disclose.

REFERENCES

1. Pribitkin E, Greywoode JD. Sonic rhinoplasty: innovative applications. Facial Plast Surg 2013;29(02): 127–32.
2. Gerbault O, Daniel RK, Kosins AM. The role of piezoelectric instrumentation in rhinoplasty surgery. Aesthet Surg J 2016;36(1):21–34.
3. Goksel A, Saban Y. Open piezo preservation rhinoplasty: a case report of the new rhinoplasty approach. Facial Plast Surg 2019; 35(01):113–8.
4. Labanca M, Azzola F, Vinci R, et al. Piezoelectric surgery: twenty years of use. Br J Oral Maxillofac Surg 2008;46(4):265–9.
5. Stoetzer M, Felgenträger D, Kampmann A, et al. Effects of a new piezoelectric device on periosteal microcirculation after subperiosteal preparation. Microvasc Res 2014;94:114–8.
6. Von See C, Gellrich NC, Rücker M, et al. Investigation of perfusion in osseous vessels in close vicinity to piezo-electric bone cutting. Br J Oral Maxillofac Surg 2012;50(3):251–5.
7. Gonzalez-Lagunas J. Is the piezoelectric device the new standard for facial osteotomies? J Stomatol Oral Maxillofac Surg 2017;118(4):255–8.
8. Tirelli G, Tofanelli M, Bullo F, et al. External osteotomy in rhinoplasty: piezosurgery vs osteotome. Am J Otol 2015;36(5):666–71.
9. Taşkın Ü, Batmaz T, Erdil M, et al. The comparison of edema and ecchymosis after piezoelectric and conventional osteotomy in rhinoplasty. Eur Arch Otorhinolaryngol 2017;274(2):861–5.
10. Robiony M, Polini F, Costa F, et al. Ultrasound piezoelectric vibrations to perform osteotomies in rhinoplasty. J Oral Maxillofac Surg 2007;65(5): 1035–8.
11. Robiony M, Lazzarotto A, Nocini R, et al. Piezosurgery: ten years' experience of percutaneous osteotomies in rhinoplasty. J Oral Maxillofac Surg 2019; 77(6):1237–44.
12. Ghassemi A, Prescher A, Talebzadeh M, et al. Osteotomy of the nasal wall using a newly designed piezo scalpel—a cadaver study. J Oral Maxillofac Surg 2013;71(12):2155.e1-e6.

13. Robotti E, Khazaal A, Leone F. Piezo-assisted turbinoplasty: a novel rapid and safe technique. Facial Plast Surg 2020;36(3):235–41.

14. Koc B, Koc EA, Erbek S. Comparison of clinical outcomes using a Piezosurgery device vs. a conventional osteotome for lateral osteotomy in rhinoplasty. Ear Nose Throat J 2017;96(8):318–26.

15. Fallahi HR, Keyhan SO, Fattahi T, et al. Comparison of piezosurgery and conventional osteotomy post rhinoplasty morbidities: a double-blind randomized controlled trial. J Oral Maxillofac Surg 2019;77(5):1050–5.

16. Troedhan A. Piezotome rhinoplasty reduces postsurgical morbidity and enhances patient satisfaction: a multidisciplinary clinical study. J Oral Maxillofac Surg 2016;74(8):1659.e1–11.

17. Pribitkin EA, Lavasani LS, Shindle C, et al. Sonic rhinoplasty: sculpting the nasal dorsum with the ultrasonic bone aspirator. Laryngoscope 2010;120(8):1504–7.

18. Mirza AA, Alandejani TA, Al-Sayed AA. Piezosurgery versus conventional osteotomy in rhinoplasty: a systematic review and meta-analysis. Laryngoscope 2020;130(5):1158–65.

19. Robiony M, Toro C, Costa F, et al. Piezosurgery: a new method for osteotomies in rhinoplasty. J Craniofac Surg 2007;18(5):1098–100.

New Concepts in Dorsal Hump Reduction

Tirbod Fattahi, MD, DDS*, Sepideh Sabooree, MD, DDS

KEYWORDS

- Hump reduction • Overprojected nose • Dorsal hump reduction

KEY POINTS

- Recognition of exact cause of a dorsal hump is critical; is it a nasal issue or a maxillary issue?
- Completion of all necessary steps in order to reduce a bony hump is very important.
- Addressing the nose following a large hump removal is imperative and must be adhered to.

INTRODUCTION

Nasal hump reduction is a commonly performed procedure in most rhinoplasties, especially in Caucasian rhinoplasty whereby overprojection of the nasal complex might be a cosmetic concern. Achieving smooth dorsal lines, a balanced nose shape, and an aesthetic transition from the nasal bridge toward the nasal tip are requirements for an ideal rhinoplasty outcome. The keystone area of the nose comprises the dorsal hump, the area where the nasal bones of the bony vault attach to the cartilaginous vault (dorsal septum and upper lateral cartilages). This osseocartilaginous junction corresponds to the rhinion anatomically. There are multiple issues that can create a true dorsal hump, or give the "illusion" of an existence of a dorsal hump. Essentially, a dorsal hump is made up of overprojected upper lateral cartilages, tall nasal bones, an overprojected dorsal septum, or a combination of the above. In this article, a brief overview of the causation of dorsal hump is presented followed by surgical options available to address this deformity. Management of the nasal dorsum following hump reduction is also highlighted.

Assessment

It is the authors' opinion that 3 distinct areas must be assessed when examining the nose from a profile view. These areas include the radix, middorsum, and the nasal tip. All 3 areas can, either independently or collectively, contribute to an actual dorsal hump or create an "illusion" of a dorsal hump.

Although there are multiple measurements, angles, and assessment tools for analyzing the objective size of an ideal nose, there is no substitute for experience and an aesthetic sense. A low radix can certainly contribute to the creation of a "pseudo-hump" as well as an underprojected or ptotic nasal tip. This is certainly highlighted when evaluating a patient for a maxillary orthognathic surgery. Patients' noses with anterior-posterior vector deficiency of the maxilla have the appearance of a large dorsal hump because of underprojection of the nasal tip. On correction of the nasal tip by advancing the anterior nasal spine during a maxillary osteotomy, the "pseudo-hump" disappears (**Figs. 1** and **2**). Oftentimes, dorsal augmentation, or appropriate tip support, as opposed to dorsal hump reduction, is what is actually necessary for some patients with a low radix or an underprojected nasal tip (**Fig. 3**).

The middorsum certainly is the main area of focus during the examination of the nose in profile. An appropriate assessment of the size of the hump and its components is critical in the preoperative period. Dorsal humps come in a variety of sizes and shapes and as aforementioned are made up of cartilage (dorsal septal cartilage, upper lateral cartilages) as well as bone (nasal bones) (**Fig. 4**).

Department of Oral & Maxillofacial Surgery, University of Florida College of Medicine, 653-1 West 8th Street, Jacksonville, FL 32209, USA
* Corresponding author.
E-mail address: Tirbod.Fattahi@Jax.Ufl.Edu

Oral Maxillofacial Surg Clin N Am 33 (2021) 31–37
https://doi.org/10.1016/j.coms.2020.09.010
1042-3699/21/© 2020 Elsevier Inc. All rights reserved.

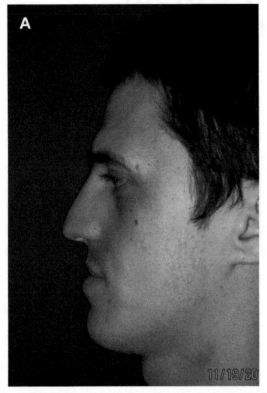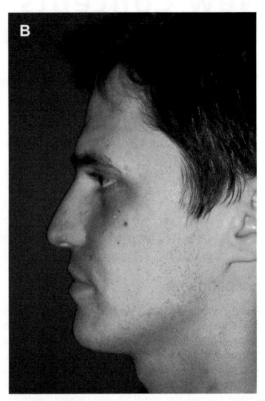

Fig. 1. (*A, B*) A "pseudo-hump" correction before and after maxillary advancement surgery. Note improvement in the nasal profile simply by repositioning of the maxilla.

Typically, there is a lateral bony extension along the dorsal sidewalls that must also be accounted for during surgery.

Surgical Considerations

Hump removal can be performed via the open structure technique (preferred method of the authors) or via the endonasal closed technique. Before the actual hump reduction, the surgeon must decide how much of the dorsum to remove

and whether to proceed with the hump reduction before or following harvesting of the septum. The actual amount of the hump reduction is really an aesthetic assessment; assuming the radix and nasal tip are supported appropriately and of adequate size, a few millimeters reduction is all that is typically necessary. Undercorrection/overcorrection of the hump can lead to deformities that would later require a revision rhinoplasty. Imbalance between resection of cartilaginous

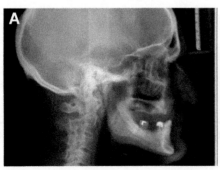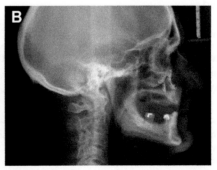

Fig. 2. (*A, B*) Preoperative and postoperative lateral radiographs demonstrating improvement in the appearance of the nasal dorsum by advancement of the maxilla.

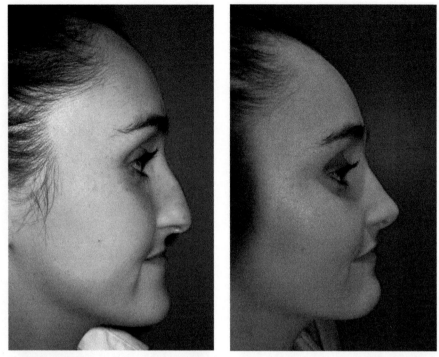

Fig. 3. Preoperative and postoperative photographs following appropriate tip support. Note improvement in nasal dorsum without any hump reduction.

part of the hump and the bony part may lead to a "pollybeak deformity."[1] It is imperative to account for the amount of hump reduction when deciding to preserve a 10-mm "L"-strut of the membranous septum. If the surgeon leaves a 10-mm L-strut and then proceeds with a 4-mm hump reduction, the remaining strut may no longer be 10 mm (as the dorsal septum usually contributes to the hump), and this could certainly lead to collapse of the

midvault. For this reason, the authors' preference is to always reduce the hump *before* any septal harvest. The authors elevate the nasal mucosa off the underside of the dorsal hump (underside of upper lateral cartilages and dorsal septum) before its resection, as it is routinely performed during a septoplasty but without actually removing the septum. Once the ideal dorsal lines have been created, then the septal harvest is begun.

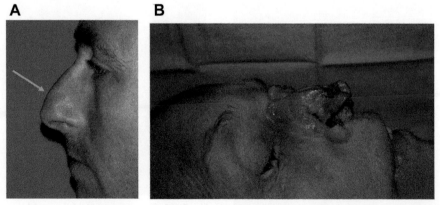

Fig. 4. (*A*) Patient with moderately sized dorsal hump. Note appropriate radix projection. Patient also demonstrates an overprojected anterior septal angle (*arrow*). (*B*) Cadaveric demonstration of a moderately sized nasal hump after removal of overlying soft tissue. Note overprojected dorsal septum, upper lateral cartilages, and nasal bones.

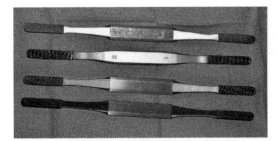

Fig. 5. Examples of nasal rasps with various coarseness.

A

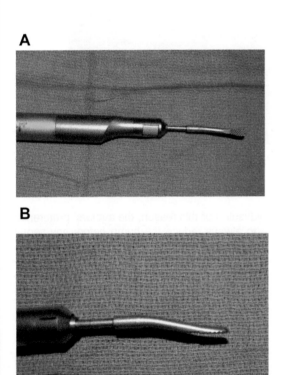

B

C

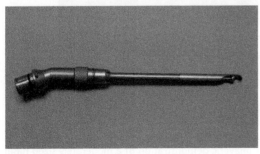

Fig. 6. Various types of power rasps (*A*, *B*) and safe-guarded drill bit (*C*) used in hump reduction.

A

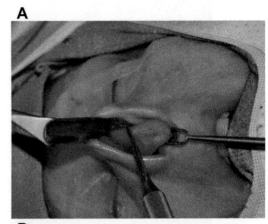

B

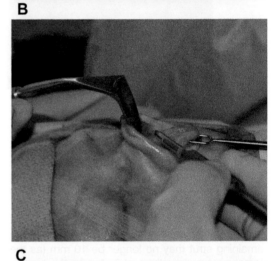

C

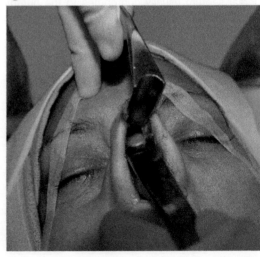

Fig. 7. (*A*, *B*) Engagement of the cartilaginous portion of the hump using a number 15 blade. (*C*) Engagement of the bony hump via a double-guarded osteotome.

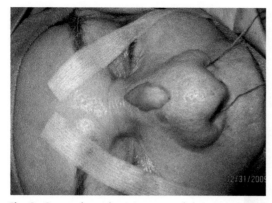

Fig. 8. Canoe-shaped appearance of the osseocartilaginous hump following removal.

Surgical Options

After appropriate exposure, the hump is visualized (via open technique), and a decision must be made regarding its management. Regardless of the technique used, it is important to reconstruct the keystone area after major hump reduction (see later discussion). A variety of options exist for management of a dorsal hump, including the following:

1. Hand-held rasps
2. Rotary instrument
   a. Traditional drills versus ultrasound drills (Piezo)
3. Blade and double-guarded osteotome
4. Push-down technique (keystone preservation technique)

Small, cartilaginous humps can easily be addressed using rasps. Rasps should be used in a pulling motion and should proceed from the most coarse to the most fine working ends (**Fig. 5**). Use of a rasp alone may lead to formation of some irregularities of the dorsum; therefore, it is important to redrape the soft tissue frequently to ensure proper reduction and avoidance of overresection.[2–7]

Rotary instruments are a quick and convenient way to address a bony dorsal hump. Some clinicians will use a rasp or a blade to resect the cartilaginous components and then switch to a surgical drill for the remaining bony portion. Most surgical drill bits have a protective sheath or are considered "safeguard" in order to avoid injuring the overlying soft tissue envelope (**Fig. 6**). Again, it is prudent to proceed judiciously and not overresect the keystone area. In recent years, Piezo surgical drills have become quite popular in maxillofacial surgery, including rhinoplasty. The key advantages of this technology are preservation of the soft tissue envelope, a more precise osteoplasty, and effortless cutting of bone because of the ultrasound waves. It is important to remember that Piezo rhinoplasty does increase the length of the operation because cutting occurs at a much slower rate and speed. Piezo surgery is discussed in another article in this issue.

Use of a number 15 blade and a double-guarded osteotome is perhaps the most traditional and tried-and-true technique in hump reduction. After proper exposure, the blade engages the soft cartilaginous portion of the hump (the most caudal edge of dorsal septal cartilage and upper lateral cartilages) and advances cephalically until meeting resistance of the nasal bones. Then a double safe-guarded osteotome is inserted into the same exact area. The osteotome is held parallel to the ideal dorsal lines and advanced until the hump is removed (**Fig. 7**). It is important to advance the soft tissue envelope over the double-guarded osteotome as it is advanced cephalically. The resection has the typical

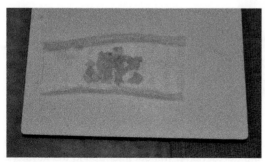

Fig. 9. Morselized and diced cartilage graft to be used for improvement of dorsal contour.

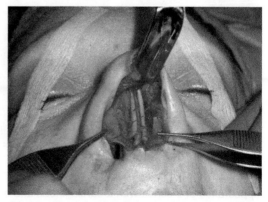

Fig. 10. Bilateral extended spreader grafts in place. Horizontal mattress sutures attach the left and right upper lateral cartilages to the grafts and the septum.

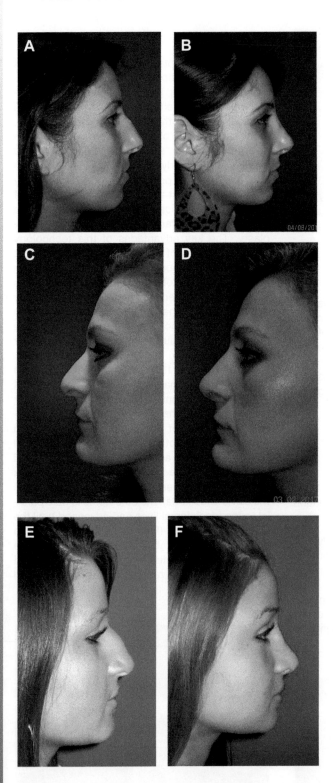

Fig. 11. (*A–F*) Preoperative and postoperative images following hump reduction and other maneuvers after an open structure rhinoplasty.

appearance of a canoe with a cartilaginous and a bony component (**Fig. 8**).

The "push-down technique" and the "let-down technique" are relatively newer procedures introduced by some investigators in order to reduce the dorsal hump without interrupting the keystone anatomy. These techniques are used to preserve the dorsal lines and to avoid collapse of the internal nasal valves.[8,9] Resection and osteotomies are made along the septum and lateral nasal walls in order to "drop" the entire nasal complex without disturbing the keystone area. The push-down operation consists of downward impaction of mobilized nasal pyramid with a high septal resection (used for smaller humps), whereas the let-down technique involves additional wedge resection of the frontal processes of the maxilla.[8] Advocates of these maneuvers tout their effectiveness; however, in the opinion of the authors, these are rather technique-sensitive procedures and not as predictable as a formal resection of the dorsal hump and appropriately reconstructing the rhinion area.

The authors' preferred sequence of maneuvers is as follows:

1. Exposure of the dorsum
2. Elevation of nasal mucosa off the underside of septum and upper lateral cartilages
3. Hump reduction
4. Harvest of septum

Post–Hump Removal Maneuvers

Regardless of the technique used, most large hump removals create an open roof deformity. Open roof deformity essentially occurs as one transforms a "dome" into a "flat ceiling." If left untreated, an open roof deformity will create a "boxy" nose that can be quite unnatural and unattractive. Bilateral lateral osteotomies must be performed in order to close the open roof deformity and recreate a dorsal dome, albeit a much smaller and smoother one. It is imperative to redrape the soft tissue and carefully palpate the underlying bony contour of the keystone area. Oftentimes, fine rasping is necessary to address surface irregularities. At times, morselized cartilage can be placed to camouflage any residual deformity (**Fig. 9**). The authors' preferred method of keystone reconstruction is to place unilateral or bilateral spreader grafts. Spreader grafts or autospreader grafts can improve breathing through enhancement of the internal nasal valves, straighten the nose, and add stability to the undermined osseocartilaginous junction. These grafts also reconstitute the attachment of the upper lateral cartilages to the nasal dorsum, thereby adding significant stability to the entire nasal complex (**Fig. 10**). The authors' preferred sequence of maneuvers following hump removal is as follows:

1. Bilateral lateral osteotomies
2. Fine rasping to ensure smooth dorsal contour
3. Placement of spreader grafts
4. Placement of morselized cartilage (if necessary) to ensure a smooth dorsal contour

5. Remaining portions of the rhinoplasty (tip work, and so forth)

SUMMARY

Dorsal hump reduction is a commonly performed maneuver in most rhinoplasty procedures. Based on the size of the hump and personal preferences, multiple options exist to address a dorsal hump. Simple rasping may be adequate for small dorsal humps, whereas newer techniques offer an alternative to the more traditional and still reliable methods. Precise adjustments must be made to avoid overcorrection/undercorrection of the hump, in order to prevent the need for a revision rhinoplasty. Regardless of the method used to remove a dorsal hump, specific attention must be paid to address the dorsum following a hump removal to ensure a functional and aesthetic outcome (**Fig. 11**).

DISCLOSURE

The authors have nothing to disclose.

REFERENCES

1. Bierenbroodspot F, et al. Dorsal hump reduction and osteotomies." Rhinoplasty Archive. 2020. Available at: www.rhinoplastyarchive.com/articles/bony-vault-nasal-dorsum/dorsal-hump-reduction.
2. Zucchini S, Brancatelli S, Piccinato A, et al. Evaluation of surgical outcome in rhinoplasty: a comparison between rasp and osteotome in dorsal hump removal. Ear Nose Throat J 2019. https://doi.org/10.1177/0145561319883529. 14556131988352.
3. Fallahi HR, Keyhan SO, Fattahi T, et al. Comparison of piezosurgery and conventional osteotomy post rhinoplasty morbidities: a double-blind randomized controlled trial. J Oral Maxillofac Surg 2019;77(5):1050–5.
4. Fattahi T. Considerations in revision rhinoplasty: lessons learned. Oral Maxillofac Surg Clin North Am 2011;23(1):101–8.
5. Fattahi T, Quereshy F. Septoplasty: thoughts and considerations. J Oral Maxillofac Surg 2011;69(12):e528–32.
6. Fallahi HR, Keyhan SO, Fattahi T, et al. Transcutaneous alar rim graft: an effective technique to manage alar deformity. J Oral Maxillofac Surg 2020;78(5):821.e1-8.
7. Fattahi T. Internal nasal valve: significance in nasal air flow. J Oral Maxillofac Surg 2008;66(9):1921–6.
8. Saban Y, Daniel RK, Polselli R, et al. Dorsal preservation: the push down technique reassessed. Aesthet Surg J 2018;38(2):117–31.
9. Gola R. Functional and esthetic rhinoplasty. Aesthetic Plast Surg 2003;27:390–6.

New Concepts in Dorsal Nasal Augmentation

Shahrokh C. Bagheri, DMD, MD[a], Behnam Bohluli, DMD, FRCD(C)[b],*,
Pouyan Sadr-Eshkevari, DMD, MD[c], Nima Moharamnejad, DMD, MD, FIBCSOMS[d]

KEYWORDS

- Dorsal augmentation • Warping • Fascia graft • Costal cartilage graft • Cartilage warping

KEY POINTS

- Autologous cartilages are commonly known as the gold standard in dorsal augmentation.
- Septal, auricular, costochondral cartilage, and temporalis fascia are common autografts for dorsal augmentation.
- Septal cartilage is ideal for minimal to moderate augmentation.
- Warping is the main limitation of costochondral graft and needs to be managed by one of the known effective techniques.
- Engineered cartilage regeneration is an emerging technique that may resolve many limitations of common grafting techniques.

INTRODUCTION

Dorsal augmentation is commonly indicated in many primary and secondary aesthetic nose surgeries. Throughout the history, various synthetic and autogenous materials have been used for dorsal augmentation. The first descriptions of dorsal augmentation dates back to late 1800 when sterile paraffin was used to augment saddle nose deformity[1,2]; surprisingly, this immature idea was widely accepted resulting in many disastrous local and systemic complications.[1,2] There are several other sporadic efforts at the same time to use bird bone, pork cartilage, and cow leather in restoring defective dorsum.[1] Jack Josef reported the first relatively successful xenografts for dorsal augmentations. He used handmade ivory implant specific for each patient to augment the nose. His brilliant handcrafts resulted in a 40% success rate.[1,3] Von Mangoldt may be considered the pioneering figure in the use of autografts for aesthetic surgery; he used the first autogenous graft to repair saddle nose in 2 cases of syphilis.[1,4] Many of the most renowned facial plastic surgeons of the time immediately followed his approach but before long, the major drawback of the application of costal cartilage revealed itself: distortion and warping.[4,5]

Gillies[4] suggested to leave a small part of perichondrium on one side of graft to control warping. Mowlem (1938) stored costochondral grafts in the abdominal wall to control distortion.[4,5] Nevertheless, none of these techniques fully prevented warping, and both Gillies and Mowlem suggested the application of bone grafts for dorsal augmentation. Tibia, calvarium, and iliac bone were commonly used for nasal augmentation but were very tough to carve and shape, resulting in very unpredictable and unsatisfactory outcomes.[5] This convinced the rhinoplastic surgeons that autogenous cartilage, with all its shortcomings, would still be the material of choice. Peer[6,7] in 1945 showed

[a] Georgia Oral and Facial Reconstructive Surgery, 4561 Olde Perimeter Way, Atlanta, GA 30346, USA;
[b] Department of Oral and Maxillofacial Surgery, University of Toronto, 124 Edward St, Toronto ON M5G 1G6, Canada; [c] School of Dentistry, University of Louisville, Room 148, 501 S. Preston Street, Louisville, Kentucky 40202, USA; [d] Department of Oral and Maxillofacial surgery, Istanbul Aydin university, Beşyol Mahallesi, İnönü Caddesi & Akasya Sk. No:6, 34295 Küçükçekmece/İstanbul, Turkey
* Corresponding author.
E-mail address: sbagher@hotmail.com

Oral Maxillofacial Surg Clin N Am 33 (2021) 39–50
https://doi.org/10.1016/j.coms.2020.09.007
1042-3699/21/© 2020 Elsevier Inc. All rights reserved.

that septal cartilage has ideal properties for nasal grafting. Later, the use of conchal cartilage proved to be efficient.[8] Surgeons, therefore, came up with novel armamentarium to harvest and prepare these grafts. All efforts have since focused on finding the best techniques to prepare and apply the cartilage graft. In this article, we give an overview of basic concepts of cartilage grafting, review new concepts of dorsal augmentation, and discuss some emerging engineering modalities.

SELECTION OF THE GRAFT SOURCE FOR DORSAL AUGMENTATION

Autogenous graft is generally accounted for as the gold standard in dorsal augmentation. Temporalis fascia, septal, auricular, and costal cartilage are the most commonly used autogenous grafts in rhinoplasty.[9–11] The choice of donor site is very determinant.[10] A comprehensive review of surgical history will reveal any possible donor site manipulations due to previous procedures. In revision rhinoplasty, septum may have been previously opened and it is recommended not to reenter the septum if there is no remaining septal deviations or spurs. Calcified rib is a common condition that is best to be detected preoperatively. A history of autoplasty would be a red flag in the choice of conchal grafts.[9,11]

The surgeon should meticulously evaluate the recipient site (nasal dorsum) preoperatively. Cartilage blocks may show a shadow of sharp edge under thin skin, while being a good choice under thicker skin. All these details should be discussed preoperatively, and consent should be taken for any possible change of plan during the operation.[9–11]

DORSAL HUMP REINSERTION, A RESCUE TECHNIQUE

In 1966, Skoog[12] presented his innovative approach in dorsal hump surgery to create a smooth dorsal contour. In this technique, first a bony-cartilaginous cap is removed from the nasal dorsum, the preplanned amount of nasal dorsum is then trimmed and removed, and finally, the hump cap is reinserted as an autograft.[12] This technique has been used for decades.[13,14] Meanwhile, in current conservative concepts of rhinoplasty, there is no tendency for these aggressive approaches, and there remain 2 relatively rare and highly resuscitative indications for this technique.

- Inadvertent hump resection: sometimes a big hump is inadvertently resected. It is very practical to trim and refine the resected hump and reinsert it instead of thinking about graft harvesting or planning a second surgery.[13,14]
- In many rhinoplasties, a combination of hump resection and radix augmentation is indicated. In these surgeries, a small cap of hump may be obtained in the routine hump surgery and used for radix augmentation[15] (**Fig. 1**).

SEPTAL CARTILAGE FOR DORSAL AUGMENTATION

Septal cartilage is an ideal material for minimal to moderate dorsal augmentations. It may be easily harvested during rhinoplasty specially when simultaneous septoplasty is to be performed.[6,7,10,11]

How much of the septal cartilage may be harvested?

Killian and Moster in 1905 emphasized that harvesting cartilage should only be done from the central part of the septum and an L-strut needs to be preserved.[16] Freer[17] suggested a minimum of 6 to 8 mm of width for the L-strut to ensure the stability of the nose (**Fig. 2**A). Surgeons have now followed these principles for a long time. Meanwhile, many later studies have shown that preservation of even 10 to 15 mm of cartilage does not guarantee nasal stability and the following parameters as well as the L-strut dimensions need to considered when septal graft harvest is planned[18–22]:

- Wide septal cartilage resections may cause small displacements of weakened septum during breathing and lead to sever nasal airway damage. Therefore, nasal airway still may be damaged despite an intact mucosa and a strong L-strut.[18]
- Ted Mau and colleagues[19] showed that leaving a triangle of cartilage in the junction of the bone and cartilage considerably increases the strength of L-strut. This may be simply done by making a back-cut in bone and cartilage junction (**Fig. 2**B).
- At least 40% of the caudal wing of the L-strut should seat on maxillary crest. It means that the protruding part of nasal cartilage that extends from anterior nasal spine (ANS) does not increase stability of L-strut. A simple guideline is to draw an imaginary line from the caudal edge of the boney vault to ANS. Harvesting may be done from back of this line (**Fig. 2**A–C).[20]
- Thickness of dorsal cartilage is much more important than the width of the L. Therefore, if dorsal cartilage is very thin, the surgeon should preserve a wider strut.[21]

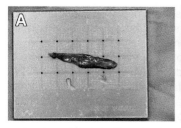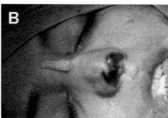

Fig. 1. (*A*) Resected hump may be tailored and (*B*) used for radix augmentation.

- Sharp angles in L-strut create internal stresses and weak points. Chamfering the right angles will remove these weak points (see **Fig. 2**C).[22]
- Conservative and reconstructive septoplasties are progressively growing.[23] Modern septoplasty usually does not advocate a large harvest of septal cartilage and rhinoplastic surgeon should justify if they want to harvest a wider septal cartilage or they rather consider other secondary donor sites.
- Cartilage crushing, cartilage dicing, or suturing several pieces together may alleviate the need for harvesting a large piece of septal cartilage.

PREPARING THE SEPTAL GRAFT FOR DORSAL AUGMENTATION
Crushed Cartilage

Crushing the cartilage graft may potentially alleviate major complications of grafting such as visible edges and graft warping.[24–26] Meanwhile, the popularity of technique has waxed and waned several times in the history of the rhinoplasty. The main challenges in using crushed cartilage have been the extent of crushing and the viabilities of the grafts.[27,28] Cakmak and colleagues[29–33] in 2005 started a series of studies that made a strong scientific backbone for this techniques and served as a guide for surgeons through most of their concerns. They proposed a classification for septal cartilage crushing that may help the surgeons plan their graft preparation for optimal results. Based on this classification, cartilage may be (1) slightly crushed, (2) moderately crushed, (3) significantly crushed, or (4) severely crushed (see **Table 1** for specifications of each class).[29] These investigators found that the vitality of cells in the crushed septal cartilage is directly related to the crushing techniques and the severity of crushing. They showed that chondrocytes retain their viability in slightly crushed and moderately crushed septal cartilages, and the percentage of viable cells is only minimally lower than the intact cartilage.[30] Another one of their studies indicated that, in the long-term follow-ups, the slightly crushed cartilages are highly predictable, whereas moderately crushed septal cartilages are more likely to result in subtle resorptions. On the other hand, the significantly crushed and the severely crushed cartilages resorbed significantly and were extremely unpredictable.[31]

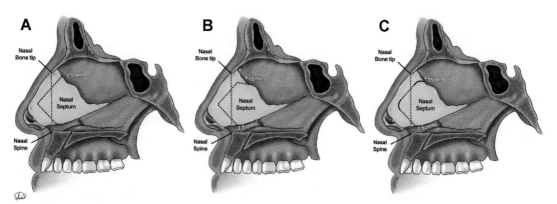

Fig. 2. (*A*) A strong L needs to be saved in septum. (*B*) A back-cut at the junction of the cartilage and bone considerably increases the strength of the nasal septum. (*C*) It is recommended to avoid sharp edges to eliminate tension zones. (*A-C*) An imaginarily line is drawn from caudal edge of the bone to the anterior nasal spine. It is recommended that the vertical wing of the L-strut to seat on the bone anterior to this line (enough width of vertical wing).

Table 1
The classification of crushed cartilages

Grade I	Slightly crushed	Moderate-force hit to soften the surface without reducing the elastic strength of the cartilage
Grade II	Moderately crushed	Moderate-force hits to soften the surface and reduce the elastic strength
Grade III	Significantly crushed	Moderate-force hits enough to cause the graft to bend with gravity
Grade IV	Severely crushed	5 or 6 forceful hits to totally destroy the integrity of the cartilage

Pearls and Pitfalls

- Nasal septal graft and auricular cartilages may be used for crushing (**Fig. 3**).
- Crushing is an extremely sensitive technique and is better to be done gently to save the viability.
- Crushed cartilage may be fixed by delicate polydioxanone sutures.
- Precision eliminates the need for overcorrection.
- Under thin skins, crushed cartilage may create sharp edges or shadows that are visible on the dorsum. Covering the crushed cartilage with a layer of fascia (sandwich technique) may be an effective solution (**Fig. 4**).[34]

Temporoparietal Fascia

Autogenous fascia especially temporoparietal fascia is commonly used in many facial cosmetic and reconstructive procedures.[9–11,35–40] Gerosantos (1984) showed versatile applications of deep temporalis fascia in a large number of rhinoplasties.[35] Daniel presented his approach in augmenting the deep radix with temporalis fascia,[36] and Daniel and Calvert[37] showed how diced cartilage wrapped in fascia may be effective in dorsal nasal augmentation. The main advantages of temporalis graft in dorsal nasal augmentation are essay access to harvest the graft, predictable long-term results and very smooth architecture that does not cause any sharp edges or shadows.[9–11] In general, the main indications of temporalis fasciae in dorsal augmentation are as follows:

- Minimal dorsal augmentation. Temporalis fascia may be spread over dorsum to minimally enhance dorsum.
- It may be rolled to make a bigger volume to augment a deep radix (**Fig. 5**).
- Temporalis fascia may be used to cover irregularities of the dorsum after using other augmentation techniques.
- Temporalis fascia may be used to wrap diced cartilages (see diced cartilage later in this article).

SURGICAL TECHNIQUE
Conventional Approach

This approach involves a 3-cm to 4-cm incision in the temporalis region, along the hair-bearing area above the ear. After locating the superficial temporal artery and vein and reaching the glistening surface of the deep temporalis fascia, a wide dissection is made to expose the donor area. Then, the graft is marked and harvested. The main drawback of this technique is the possibility of hair loss in incision lines. However, with precise incisions parallels with hair follicles, meticulous surgical techniques and appropriate wound closure, incision line would be adequately concealed by hair.[38,39]

Neck Hairline Approach

In this approach, a 3-cm to 5-cm curvilinear incision is made at the neck hairline. After finding the surgical plane, access to the deep temporalis fasciae is obtained by dissecting upward and forward. Incision line is concealed, and there is little or no risk of hair follicle damage. Moreover, the incision may be used for simultaneous access to mastoid fascia when more graft material is needed (see **Fig. 4**A, B; **Fig. 6**).[40]

Miscellaneous Fascial Tissues

There has been a growing interest in using different fasciae in rhinoplasty. Postauricular fascia,[41,42] mastoid fascia,[43,44] fascia lata,[45,46] pectorals major fascia,[47] rectus muscle fascia,[48] precranial fasciae,[49] and rectus abdomens fascia[50] are reported to have different indications for dorsal augmentation. Ease of access, possible complications, surgeon's skills and experience, patient's compliance, and more importantly the strength of evidence in support of each technique will dictate the choice of the best fascial material for any specific case. **Table 2** presents a summary of some of the most common fascial grafts and their use in dorsal nasal augmentation.

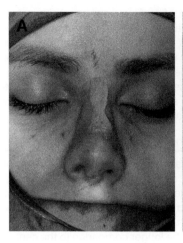
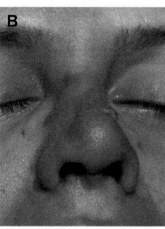

Fig. 3. (*A, B*) Crushed cartilage is a feasible graft for minimal dorsal augmentation.

Costochondral Graft for Dorsal Augmentation

Costochondral graft provides a considerable amount of cartilage that may be used for structural reconstruction of the nose.[51] Any of the ribs 5 to 11 may donate based on the indications. Donor site complications are extensively discussed in the literature. Pneumothorax, pleural tear, visible scar, and pain are the possible donor site complications. However, when properly performed, this modality is quite safe and predictable.[52,53] The main challenge in rib cartilage grafting is possible distortion.[5,52,53] There are numerous techniques to overcome this limitation.[5,37,54–60]

Warping of the Costochondral Graft

Graft distortion or warping is a frustrating complication of costochondral grafting. It may happen at any point from immediately after cutting the

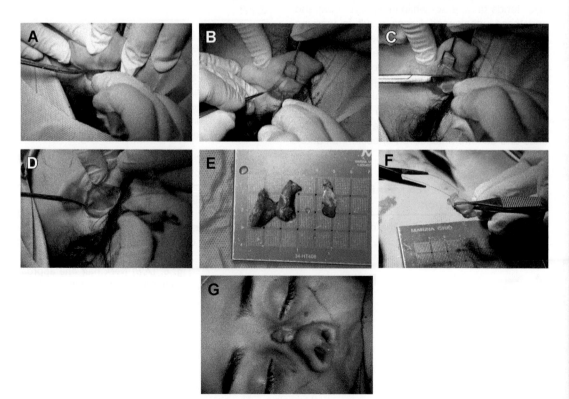

Fig. 4. (*A–C*) Graft harvest from posterior approach. (*D, E*) Mastoid fascia harvest. (*F, G*) Preparation of fascia overlying crushed cartilage (sandwich technique).

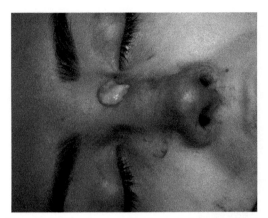

Fig. 5. Fascia is an ideal material for radix augmentation.

cartilage to many years after completion of rhinoplasty.[5,54] Gibson and Davis[5] did a comprehensive work on cartilage warping in 1965, which is still the main reference to describe and manage this phenomenon. They showed that in a rib cartilage, the superficial layer has flatter chondrocytes and a different matrix (proteoglycan proteins) comparing to the central parts of the rib.[5] The difference in layers bears a tension that in a normal nonharvested rib is neutralized by counteracting forces. After carving the harvested rib, the outer layer tends to contract while inner layers expand, and these unbalanced forces result in warping. Based on this explanation,[5] they proposed a balanced cross-section technique to avoid warping. In this method, cartilage carving is planned in a way that intrinsic opposing forces are neutralized.[5] There are many other techniques described to prevent cartilage warping. An aesthetic nose surgeon should be familiar with the most important ones and use them based on specific indications and preferences.

TECHNIQUES TO PREVENT WARPING
Balanced Cross Section

This method should equalize the opposing forces on each side of the graft (**Fig. 7**). For instance, if

there are 2 mm of surface cartilage on one side, exactly the same amount should remain on the other side. This methods relies on neutralizing of possible forces by the same amount of the force on the other side. **Fig. 5** shows some possible designs for balanced cross section. In contrast, if the carving creates any unopposed forces on the surface, it is unbalanced and unsafe (**Fig. 8**).[5]

Concentric Carving of the Rib Cartilage

Many studies have shown that peripheral parts of costal cartilage are more susceptible to warping. Harris and colleagues demonstrated that if the graft is prepared from peripheral surfaces of costal cartilage, it is 2 times more likely to warp, and this warpage would be longer comparing to the central cut pieces.[5,54–57] These findings led to the advent of a technique that aims to prepare the graft from central core of the rib cartilage[55] (see **Fig. 7C**).

Soaking in Hypertonic/Hypotonic Solutions

It is a common practice to soak harvested rib temporarily in hyper-/hypotonic solutions to prevent or control future warping. Harris and colleagues[54] showed that this treatment does not affect the process of warping.

Intraoperative Delay Before Applying the Graft

Many studies show that warping may start immediately after removing the cartilages grafts. Thus, it is feasible to harvest and carve the costochondral graft first then delay placing it on the recipient bed until the surgeon is skeletonizing the nose and performing the preliminary tip plasty. The costal cartilage will undergo its possible immediate warping and will be ready for dorsal augmentation.[54]

Mechanical Reinforcement of Costochondral Cartilage

Some investigators have tried to reinforce the cartilage and prevent warping. Gunter and colleagues[58] presented a reinforcement technique in using costal cartilage for dorsal augmentation.

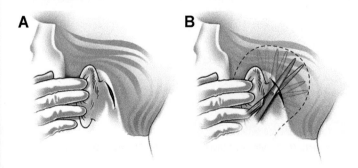

A **B**

Fig. 6. (*A, B*) Neck hair line approach to harvest temporalis fascia.

Table 2
Most common fascial grafts and their use in dorsal nasal augmentation

Fascia Donor Site	Author, Publication Year	Study Type and No. Cases	Application	Follow-Ups Months
Postauricular	Antohi et al,[42] 2012	Case series No: 16	Wrapped crushed conchal cartilage	23.1
Postauricular	Hodgkinson et al,[41] 2017	Case reports No: 3	Single graft	-
Mastoid	Dogan & Aydin,[44] 2012	Retrospective case series No: 30	Single graft	29.2
Mastoid	Hong et al,[43] 2012	Prospective case series No: 33	Wrapped diced conchal cartilage	-
Fascia lata	Karaaltin et al,[46] 2009	Retrospective case series No: 63	Single graft	20
Fascia lata	Kim et al,[55] 2011	Case report	Wrapped diced costal cartilage	14
Pectoralis major	Xavier,[47] 2015	Case reports No: 2	Wrapped diced costal cartilage	12
Rectus muscle	As'adi et al,[48] 2014	Randomized clinical trial No: 36	Wrapped diced costal cartilage with temporalis vs rectus muscle fascia	12
Pericranial	Lee et al,[51] 2019	Technical note on a trauma case	Wrapped diced conchal cartilage	-
Rectus abdominis	Cerkes & Basaran,[50] 2016	Retrospective case series No: 109	Wrapped diced costal cartilage	19.6

They inserted a Kirschner wire inside the graft to support the costal cartilage and prevent warping.[58] Oksuz and colleagues[59] adapted and fixed a miniplate under costal cartilage to help fix the graft over the dorsum and to prevent it from warping. Although these techniques have shown efficacy in controlling cartilage distortion, their popularity is hindered by the possibility of

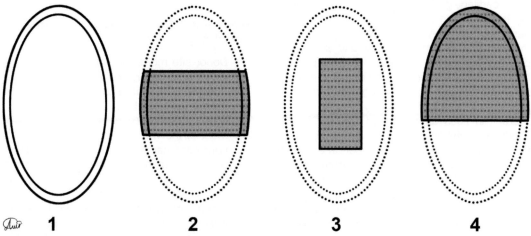

Fig. 7. Some samples of balanced preparation of the costal cartilage. (*A*) Intact cartilage. (*B–D*) Balanced carving. (*Adapted from* Gibson T, Davis WB. The distortion of autogenous cartilage grafts: its cause and prevention. Br J Plast Surg. 1958;10:263; with permission.)

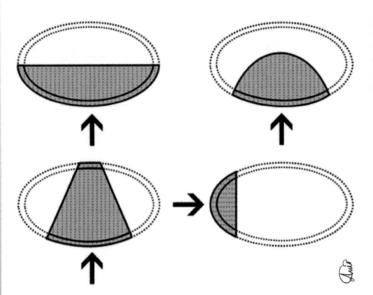

Fig. 8. Unbalanced forces cartilage will warp toward the arrow. (*Adapted from* Gibson T, Davis WB. The distortion of autogenous cartilage grafts: its cause and prevention. Br J Plast Surg. 1958;10:264; with permission.)

extrusion, possibility of infection, and a lower tendency to use foreign materials inside the nose.

Cartilage Warp Suture

Guyuron and colleagues[60] proposed the warp control suture. In this technique, a harvested rib cartilage is precisely carved to the desired shape and is then soaked for 15 minutes in normal saline to reveal any warp tendencies. Finally, the surgeon places several through and through mattress sutures from the convex part to the concave part and tighten until the distorted graft is straightened. The straightened cartilage is then used for dorsal augmentation.[60]

Diced Cartilage Graft

Diced cartilage graft is one the oldest known grafting techniques in rhinoplasty. In 1943, Peer[61,62] described his technique in cutting rib cartilage to many small (1 to 3 mm) particles and using these particles to fill and augment defective parts of the nose. Many surgeons found it hard to manipulate and introduce diced cartilages and this technique was overlooked for a long time.

Erol[63] in 2000 demonstrated an easy way to handle and use diced cartilage. In his technique, finely chopped cartilage is wrapped in a layer of absorbable Surgicel and the packed graft is simply transferred to the defective site. His article is one of the mostly cited studies in the rhinoplasty literature[64] and though it is rarely used today, it makes the backbone of many popular and effective techniques in current rhinoplasty.

The first modification was done by Daniel and Calvert.[37] They noticed that diced cartilage wrapped in Surgicel undergoes unpredictable resorption and started to wrap the diced cartilages in temporalis fascia.[37] In this technique, first the temporalis fascia is harvested; then the cartilage is finely diced into 1-mm particles; the fascia is then sutured around a 1-mL insulin syringe; the diced cartilage is filled inside the syringe; and the diced cartilage is transferred to fascial bag by pressing the plunger. This fascial bag is used as an autograft to augment the nasal dorsum (**Fig. 9A–H**). There are numerous other modifications to this technique but in general the main efforts are either to wrap the diced cartilage in different layers or to use glues or biomaterials to make a formable and easier-to-handle paste of the diced cartilage without wrapping.[65–70]

Pearls and Pitfalls in Using Costal Cartilage for Dorsal Augmentation

- Donor site morbidity would be little to none with the use of precise standard techniques.
- Surgeon should have cartilage deformation in mind preoperatively and manage it intraoperatively.
- Most of the warping happens in first half an hour after harvest; therefore, it is logical to delay placement of the graft for 30 minutes.
- Diced cartilage may solve many limitations of costal cartilage grafts.
- Diced cartilage may be wrapped in fascia to provide better control before placement; it may also be assembled by fiber glue or biological adhesives before being transferred to the dorsum.

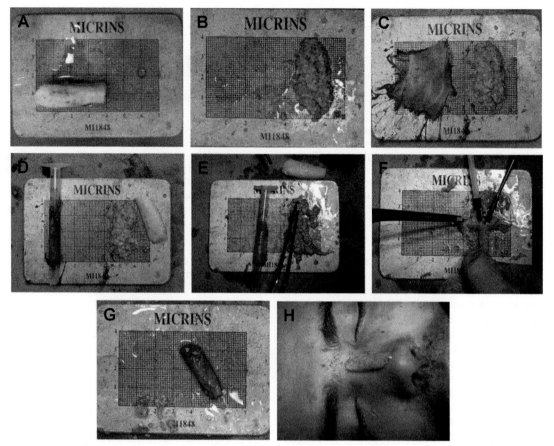

Fig. 9. (*A–H*) Different steps of providing diced cartilage wrapped on temporalis fascia.

- Despite the many advantages of diced cartilage, chopping the rib cartilage attenuates its mechanical properties.

Auricular Cartilage for Dorsal Nasal Augmentation

Ear cartilage is very accessible source of autogenous graft. Conchal cartilages is the most common site of ear for graft harvesting.[9–11,65] It provides approximately 3.84 cm of cartilage and the donor site usually heals with a very low rate of complications.[65] The main limitation of conchal cartilage is in its inherent anatomic curvatures and lower mechanical strength, which make it less desirable for major structural reconstructions. Meanwhile, common cartilage processing techniques such as slightly crushing and dicing (with or without a fasciae wrapping) make it a reasonable approach in many dorsal augmentation cases. Conchal cartilages may be harvested through anterior or posterior approaches.[9–11,65] Anterior approach has easier access and provides a smooth surface of curved cartilage. In posterior approach, the incision line is completely hidden in post auricular creas.[10]

Also it provides 2 times the amount of cartilage. Moreover, a recently described advantage is the simultaneous access to the mastoid fasciae, which may be needed in some cases.[11]

CARTILAGE BIOENGINEERING FOR DORSAL AUGMENTATION

Cartilage tissue engineering is an emerging approach to restore damaged and defective cartilages.[66,67] Cartilage is an avascular tissue which consists of only one type of cells: chondrocytes. Therefore, nasal cartilage should theoretically be tissue engineered rather simply.[67] The traditional process of cartilage engineering includes 3 basic steps. First, a small piece of cartilage is harvested by taking a sample from the patient (biopsy from nasal septum, auricular or rib cartilage); then, the cells are transferred to a 3-dimensional scaffold to increase the number of chondrocytes in a desired framework; and finally, the engineered cartilage is used as the donor and grafted to the recipient bed (**Fig. 10**).

Yanaga and colleagues[69] used auricular cartilage to generate cartilaginous tissue. They

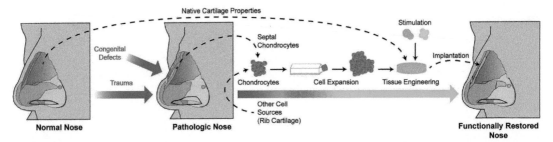

Fig. 10. Overview of nasal tissue-engineering. Chondrocytes sourced from the nasal septum or rib cartilage may be expanded and used to fabricate engineered neocartilage. Engineered neocartilage may then be implanted into a patient to correct nasal cartilage pathologies and restore functionality. To strive for biomimicry, the properties of native nasal cartilages should be used as gold standards when applying engineering strategies. (*From* Lavernia L, Brown WE, Wong BJF, et al. Toward tissue-engineering of nasal cartilages. Acta Biomater 2019;88:50; with permission.)

harvested 1 cm of auricular cartilage and extracted chondrocytes from this samples. After culturing the chondrocytes, they obtained a gelatinous immature cartilaginous tissue and injected it subcutaneously for dorsal augmentation. They reported successful dorsal augmented in 75 patients.[69] Jodat and colleagues[70] used a 3-dimensional printed scaffold made by bioinks. This innovation has helped the surgeons to receive a graft that has the exact architecture of the defective part of the nose. Cartilage tissue engineering is a promising technology that may potentially solve many grafting problems although there are still some challenges to be resolved before its widespread use.

PEARLS AND PITFALLS IN NASAL CARTILAGE ENGINEERING

- One cubic centimeter of cartilage biopsy may help produce several times the volume of similar cartilage, which would be enough for nasal augmentation.
- Donor site morbidity is considerably diminished or totally eliminated.
- Tissue engineering would be a very promising alternative in patients with a previous harvest of septal cartilage and calcified ribs.
- Mature chondrocytes that are retrieved by biopsy may undergo dedifferentiation and turn into fibroblasts or undergo overdifferentiation and turn into bone; therefore, the final tissue would not be optimal in some situations.
- Injectable tissue-engineered cartilage has been reported to be successfully used for dorsal augmentation. It is believed that injected tissue turns into rigid mature cartilage in 3 to 4 weeks.
- Stem cells are other options for cartilage engineering, but uncontrolled or unpredictable

growth of cells may end in unacceptable contour or formation of teratomas.

DISCLOSURE

The authors have nothing to disclose.

REFERENCES

1. Lupo G. The history of aesthetic rhinoplasty: special emphasis on the saddle nose. Aesthet Plast Surg 1997;21(5):309–27.
2. Goldwyn RM. The paraffin story. Plast Reconstr Surg 1980;65(4):517–24.
3. Safian J. Progress in nasal and chin augmentation. Plast Reconstr Surg 1966;37(5):446–52.
4. Gillies HD. Plastic surgery of the face. London: Oxford University Press; 1920.
5. Gibson T, Davis WB. The distortion of autogenous cartilage grafts: its cause and prevention. Br J Plast Surg 1958;10:257–73.
6. Peer LA. The neglected septal cartilage graft, with experimental observations on the growth of human cartilage grafts. Arch Otolaryngol 1945;42:384–96.
7. Peer LA. Cartilage grafting. Br J Plast Surg 1954; 7(3):250–62.
8. Stark RB, Frileck SP. Conchal cartilage grafts in augmentation rhinoplasty and orbital floor fracture. Plast Reconstr Surg 1969;43(6):591–6.
9. Bohluli B. Esthetic rhinoplasty in the multiply operated nose. J Oral Maxillofac Surg 2019;77(7):1466. e1–13.
10. Bohluli B, Varedi P. 2015. Advanced rhinoplasty: problems and solutions, a textbook of advanced oral and maxillofacial surgery Volume 2, Mohammad Hosein Kalantar Motamedi, IntechOpen, https://doi.org/10.5772/59745.
11. Bohluli B, Bagheri SC. Chapter 104: revision rhinoplasty. Current therapy in oral and maxillofacial surgery. W.B. Saunders; 2012. p. 901–10.

12. Skoog T. A method of hump reduction in rhinoplasty. a technique for preservation of the nasal roof. Arch Otolaryngol 1966;83(3):283–7.

13. Regnault P, Alfaro A. The Skoog rhinoplasty: a modified technique. Plast Reconstr Surg 1980;66(4):578–90.

14. Niechajev I. Skoog rhinoplasty revisited. Aesthet Plast Surg 2011;35(5):808–13.

15. Bohluli B, Varedi P, Bagheri SC, et al. Nasal radix augmentation in rhinoplasty: suggestion of an algorithm. Int J Oral Maxillofac Surg 2017;46(1):41–5.

16. Killlan G, Foster EE. XXIII. The submucous window resection of the nasal septum. Ann Otology, Rhinology Laryngol 1905;14(2):363–93.

17. Freer OT. The correction of deflections of the nasal septum with a minimum of traumatism. JAMA 1902;XXXVIII(10):636–42.

18. Gaball C, Lovald S, Khraishi T, et al. Engineering analysis of an unreported complication of septoplasty. Arch Facial Plast Surg 2010;12(6):385–92.

19. Mau T, Mau ST, Kim DW. Cadaveric and engineering analysis of the septal L-strut. Laryngoscope 2007;117(11):1902-6.

20. Lee JS, Lee DC, Ha DH, et al. Redefining the septal L-strut to prevent collapse. PLoS One 2016;11(4):e0153056.

21. Liu YF, Messinger K, Inman JC. Yield strength testing in human cadaver nasal septal cartilage and L-strut constructs. JAMA Facial Plast Surg 2017;19(1):40–5.

22. Glass GE, Staruch RMT, Ruston J, et al. Beyond the L-strut: redefining the biomechanics of rhinoplasty using topographic optimization modeling. Aesthet Surg J 2019;39(12):1309–18.

23. Aaronson NL, Vining EM. Correction of the deviated septum: from ancient Egypt to the endoscopic era. Int Forum Allergy Rhinol 2014;4:931–6.

24. Stoksted P, Ladefoged C. Crushed cartilage in nasal reconstruction. J Laryngol Otol 1986;100(8):897–906.

25. Collawn SS, Fix RJ, Moore JR, et al. Nasal cartilage grafts: more than a decade of experience. Plast Reconstr Surg 1997;100(6):1547–52.

26. Hamra ST. Crushed cartilage grafts over alar dome reduction in open rhinoplasty. Plast Reconstr Surg 2000;105:792–5.

27. Bujía J. Determination of the viability of crushed cartilage grafts: clinical implications for wound healing in nasal surgery. Ann Plast Surg 1994;32(3):261–5.

28. Verwoerd-Verhoef HL, Meeuwis CA, van der Heul RO, et al. Histologic evaluation of crushed cartilage grafts in the growing nasal septum of young rabbits. ORL J Otorhinolaryngol Relat Spec 1991;53(5):305–9.

29. Cakmak O, Altintas H. A classification for degree of crushed cartilage. Arch Facial Plast Surg 2010;12(6):435–6.

30. Cakmak O, Buyuklu F, Yilmaz Z, et al. Viability of cultured human nasal septum chondrocytes after crushing. Arch Facial Plast Surg 2005;7(6):406–9.

31. Cakmak O, Bircan S, Buyuklu F, et al. Viability of crushed and diced cartilage grafts: a study in rabbits. Arch Facial Plast Surg 2005;7(1):21–6.

32. Cakmak O. Crushed cartilage grafts: is overcorrection necessary? Arch Facial Plast Surg 2008;10(6):428.

33. Cakmak O, Buyuklu F. Crushed cartilage grafts for concealing irregularities in rhinoplasty. Arch Facial Plast Surg 2007;9(5):352–7.

34. Varedi P, Bohluli B. Dorsal nasal augmentation: is the composite graft consisting of conchal cartilage and retroauricular fascia an effective option? J Oral Maxillofac Surg 2015;73(9):1842.e1–13.

35. Guerrerosantos J. Temporoparietal free fascia grafts in rhinoplasty. Plast Reconstr Surg 1984;74(4):465–75.

36. Daniel RK. Mastering Rhinoplasty: A Comprehensive Atlas of Surgical Techniques.

37. Daniel RK, Calvert JW. Diced cartilage grafts in rhinoplasty surgery. Plast Reconstr Surg 2004;113(7):2156–71.

38. Besharatizadeh R, Ozkan BT, Tabrizi R. Complete or a partial sheet of deep temporal fascial graft as a radix graft for radix augmentation. Eur Arch Otorhinolaryngol 2011;268(10):1449–53.

39. Park SW, Kim JH, Choi CY, et al. Various applications of deep temporal fascia in rhinoplasty. Yonsei Med J 2015;56(1):167–74.

40. Nazari S, Bohluli B, Besharatizadeh R, et al. Neck hairline incision for simultaneous harvesting of temporal and mastoid fasciae: a technical note. J Oral Maxillofac Surg 2013;71(9):1598–600.

41. Hodgkinson DJ, Valente PM. The versatile posterior auricular fascia in secondary rhinoplasty procedures. Aesthet Plast Surg 2017;41(4):893–7.

42. Antohi N, Isac C, Stan V, et al. Dorsal nasal augmentation with "open sandwich" graft consisting of conchal cartilage and retroauricular fascia. Aesthet Surg J 2012;32(7):833–45.

43. Hong ST, Kim DW, Yoon ES, et al. Superficial mastoid fascia as an accessible donor for various augmentations in Asian rhinoplasty. J Plast Reconstr Aesthet Surg 2012;65(8):1035–40.

44. Dogan T, Aydin HU. Mastoid fascia tissue as a graft for restoration of nasal contour deformities. J Craniofac Surg 2012;23(4):e314–6.

45. Kim YH, Kim JT. Nasal reconstruction with double-layer tensor fascia lata-wrapped diced rib cartilage in a patient with severe dorsal collapse. J Craniofac Surg 2011;22(2):628–30.

46. Karaaltin MV, Orhan KS, Demirel T. Fascia lata graft for nasal dorsal contouring in rhinoplasty. J Plast Reconstr Aesthet Surg 2009;62(10):1255–60.

47. Xavier R. Pectoralis major fascia in rhinoplasty. Aesthet Plast Surg 2015;39(3):300–5.

48. As'adi K, Salehi SH, Shoar S. Rib diced cartilage-fascia grafting in dorsal nasal reconstruction: a randomized clinical trial of wrapping with rectus muscle fascia vs deep temporal fascia. Aesthet Surg J 2014;34(6):21–31.

49. Lee JT, Lee H, Yap YL, et al. A new variant of dorsal nasal graft: diced cartilage in pericranial fascia. Plast Reconstr Surg 2019;144(5):951e–2e.

50. Cerkes N, Basaran K. Diced cartilage grafts wrapped in rectus abdominis fascia for nasal dorsum augmentation. Plast Reconstr Surg 2016;137(1): 43–51.

51. Lee LN, Quatela O, Bhattacharyya N. The epidemiology of autologous tissue grafting in primary and revision rhinoplasty. Laryngoscope 2019;129(7): 1549–53.

52. Varadharajan K, Sethukumar P, Anwar M, et al. Complications associated with the use of autologous costal cartilage in rhinoplasty: a systematic review. Aesthet Surg J 2015;35(6):644–52.

53. Wee JH, Park MH, Oh S, et al. Complications associated with autologous rib cartilage use in rhinoplasty: a meta-analysis. JAMA Facial Plast Surg 2015;17(1):49–55.

54. Harris S, Pan Y, Peterson R, et al. Cartilage warping: an experimental model. Plast Reconstr Surg 1993; 92(5):912–5.

55. Kim DW, Shah AR, Toriumi DM. Concentric and eccentric carved costal cartilage: a comparison of warping. Arch Facial Plast Surg 2006;8(1):42–6.

56. Farkas JP, Lee MR, Lakianhi C, et al. Effects of carving plane, level of harvest, and oppositional suturing techniques on costal cartilage warping. Plast Reconstr Surg 2013;132(2):319–25.

57. Adams WP Jr, Rohrich RJ, Gunter JP, et al. The rate of warping in irradiated and nonirradiated homograft rib cartilage: a controlled comparison and clinical implications. Plast Reconstr Surg 1999;103(1): 265–70.

58. Gunter JP, Clark CP, Friedman RM. Internal stabilization of autogenous rib cartilage grafts in rhinoplasty: a barrier to cartilage warping. Plast Reconstr Surg 1997;100(1):161–9.

59. Eren F, Öksüz S, Melikoğlu C, et al. Saddle-nose deformity repair with microplate-adapted costal cartilage. Aesthet Plast Surg 2014;38(4):733–41.

60. Guyuron B, Wang DZ, Kurlander DE. The cartilage warp prevention suture. Aesthet Plast Surg 2018; 42(3):854–8.

61. Peer LA. Extended use of diced cartilage grafts. Plast Reconstr Surg 1954;14(3):178–85.

62. Peer LA. Diced cartilage grafts. J Int Coll Surg 1954; 22(3 Pt 1):283–91.

63. Erol OO. The Turkish delight: a pliable graft for rhinoplasty. Plast Reconstr Surg 2000;105(6):2229–41.

64. Sinha Y, Iqbal FM, Spence JN, et al. A bibliometric analysis of the 100 most-cited articles in rhinoplasty. Plast Reconstr Surg Glob Open 2016;4(7):e820.

65. Ho TT, Cochran T, Sykes KJ, et al. Costal and auricular cartilage grafts for nasal reconstruction: an anatomic analysis. Ann Otol Rhinol Laryngol 2017; 126(10):706–11.

66. Oseni AO, Butler PE, Seifalian AM. Nasal reconstruction using tissue engineered constructs: an update. Ann Plast Surg 2013;71(2):238–44.

67. Oseni A, Crowley C, Lowdell M, et al. Advancing nasal reconstructive surgery: the application of tissue engineering technology. J Tissue Eng Regen Med 2012;6(10):757–68.

68. Lavernia L, Brown WE, Wong BJF, et al. Toward tissue-engineering of nasal cartilages. Acta Biomater 2019;88:42–56.

69. Yanaga H, Imai K, Yanaga K. Generative surgery of cultured autologous auricular chondrocytes for nasal augmentation. Aesthetic Plast Surg 2009; 33(6):795-802.

70. Jodat YA, Kiaee K, Vela Jarquin D, et al. A 3D-printed hybrid nasal cartilage with functional electronic olfaction. Adv Sci (Weinh) 2020;7(5):1901878.

Preservation Dorsal Hump Surgery: A Changing Paradigm

Seied Omid Keyhan, DDS, OMFS[a,1], Behnam Bohluli, DMD, FRCD(C)[b,*], Shahriar Nazari, MD[c], Shohreh Ghasemi, DMD[d,2]

KEYWORDS

- Preservative rhinoplasty • Keystone • Soft tissue envelope • Nasal ligaments
- Push-down technique • Let-down technique

KEY POINTS

- Preservative dorsal hump surgery is an old approach that has revitalized recently.
- Preservation rhinoplasty aims to shape the existing structures instead of resection/reconstruction approaches.
- A thorough understanding of the applied anatomy of the nose is the backbone of preservative hump surgery.
- There are few techniques for preservative hump surgery, but the mainstay is to remove a strip from the septum, then to reset the osteocartilaginous vault in a lower position.
- In preservative hump surgery, keystone works as a joint, and by lowering this joint, the hump is eliminated.
- The preservative technique may facilitate simultaneous orthognathic and rhinoplasty.

INTRODUCTION

Historically dorsal hump surgery has been a smooth and very unequivocal step in rhinoplasty, and for a long time, Josef's reductive technique[1] and later Sheens reductive/reconstructive approach[2,3] have been the gold standard in dorsal hump surger.[4] Although these traditional approaches have shown to be effective in many long-term follow-ups, it is frequently shown that this approach may need a revision in 10% to 15% of cases.[5–7] This secondary surgery may be a subtle touch-up or a major reconstruction surgery with rib, conchal cartilage, and/or fasciae grafts, which will be a big challenge for both the aesthetic surgeon and rhinoplasty patient.[8,9]

New anatomic findings may be the other main reason for rethinking about dorsal hump surgery. Soft tissue envelope and osteocartilaginous vault have been comprehensively evaluated during the past decade. Soft tissue envelope is shown to be more than a simple cover of the nose. It consists of skin, subcutaneous tissue, the superficial musculoaponeurotic system (SMAS), blood vessels, and nasal ligaments. The SMAS is shown to be a continuous layer from the glabella to the nasal tip. The nasal ligaments have been shown to have a determinant role in stabilizing the anatomic element and transferring the muscular function.[10–12] Keystone has been shown as a complex anatomic structure that is very difficult or sometimes impossible to reconstruct.[13]

[a] Cranio-Maxillo-Facial Research Center for Craniofacial Reconstruction, Tehran University of Medical Sciences, Shariati Hospital, Tehran, Iran; [b] Oral and Maxillofacial Surgery, University of Toronto, 124 Edward St, Toronto, ON M5G 1G6, Canada; [c] Private practice, 154 africa (jordan st.), Tehran, Iran; [d] Department of oral and maxillofacial, University of Augusta, GA, USA

[1] Present address: Unit #3, Floor 1, Mahtab Building, Mahtab Alley, Shahid Ebrahimzadeh (#11) Alley, West Hasht-Behesht ST, Bozorgmehr ST, Isfahan 8154748915, Iran
[2] Present address: 407 bridle path, Marietta,30068 GA, USA
* Corresponding author.
E-mail address: bbohluli@yahoo.com

Oral Maxillofacial Surg Clin N Am 33 (2021) 51–59
https://doi.org/10.1016/j.coms.2020.09.013

As a result, many rhinoplasty surgeons tried to reassess preservative dorsal hump surgery techniques that were mostly overlooked in rhinoplasty literature. These rhinoplasty surgeons believe that by preserving the structure of the dorsum many of these potential problems may be avoided.[14,15] They advocate preservative techniques to bring down the existing dorsum instead of resection of the excessive part, and in this way, the convex contour (nasal hump) is corrected. In fact, preservative techniques aim to eliminate the destruction-reconstruction cycle that happens in conventional hump reduction.[15]

This article provides an overview of related literature. History of the preservation dorsal surgery, current trends, and future perspectives are discussed. It is attempted to provide practice recommendations and key points where indicated.

HISTORY

Daniel in 2018[15] proposed the term *preservation rhinoplasty* that may be a turning point in rhinoplasty to bring many sporadic rhinoplasty findings under one umbrella.

Surprisingly, the first documented preservation hump surgery dates back to 1899 when Goodale reported his technique in treating an exaggerated Roman nose (big hump) in a 13-year-old girl (**Fig. 1**).[16]

In this case, by performing 2 incisions on the nasal septum, a subdorsal strip of the cartilage and bone was removed. Then, after doing lateral osteotomies on the bony vault by nasal saws, the nasal bridge was pressed done and the excessive hump was eliminated. It is noteworthy that the nasal patency was not affected by this procedure.[16] This technique was modified and developed by Cottle in 1954.[17,18] The method is currently growing very fast, known as the *push-down* technique.

Lothrop in 1914[19] described another approach and designed a bone-cutting forceps for his technique. In his technique, a stripe of subdorsal cartilage is removed (similar to Goodale's approach) (**Fig. 2**A), then a bony wedge is resected from the nasofacial junction on both sides of the bony vault (**Fig. 2**B and C), and finally by doing a transverse osteotomy at radix, whole bony vault is pressed down and the excessive hump is eliminated (**Fig. 3**). Lothrop was surprised that despite creating a smaller nose, airway was improved after this procedure. This technique is frequently modified, but the general concept is commonly used in modern rhinoplasty and is known as *let-down* procedure.

Despite some well-executed studies such as that by Jammet and colleagues in 1989[20] on 87 patients and Ishida's comprehensive report on 125 patients (1999)[21] that demonstrated the potentials of preservative techniques, these brilliant pioneer works have been mostly overlooked for a long time in favor of Josef's reductive techniques. Saban and his colleagues reported their extensive work on the soft tissue envelope of the nose. They showed that the nasal SMAS extends from glabella to nasal tip and particular regions give few ligamentous extensions that these ligaments transfer the functions of the nasal muscles to the osteocartilaginous framework of the nose.

Therefore, mechanical reconstruction of the nose by spreader grafts will not restore the whole internal nasal valve functioning.[10] Cakir proposed subperichondrial/subperiosteal dissections to save the integrity of nasal ligaments and minimize the trauma to soft tissue components such as nerves, vessels, and muscle.[12]

Saban and colleagues had a dominant role in the repopularization of the preservative techniques. They reassessed the push-down and let-down techniques and demonstrated a very

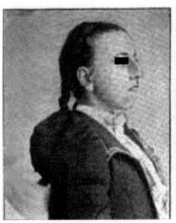 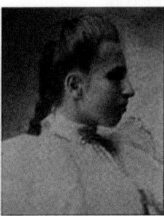

Fig. 1. (*A, B*) Goodale's case, treated with push-down technique. (*From* Goodale JL. A new method for the operative correction of exaggerated roman nose. Boston Med Surg J. 1899;140:112.)

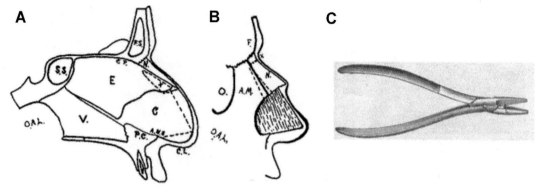

Fig. 2. (*A–C*) Lothrop's techniques for hump surgery. (*A*) Subdorsal septal resection. (*B*) Bony wedge resection. (*C*) Lathrop's forceps for bone resection. (*From* Lothrop OA. An operation for correcting the aquiline nasal deformity; the use of new instrument; report of a case. Boston Med Surg J. 1914;170:835–7.)

practical modification that solved most complexities of the original Cottle's technique.[14]

Kosins (2020) performed a comprehensive review of his cases and classified common indications and approaches and showed how the proper treatment plan may alleviate some limitations of preservative hump surgery and add indications that were excluded from these approaches beforehand.[22]

APPLIED ANATOMY
Soft Tissue Envelope

The soft tissue of the nose encompasses several distinct layers. The SMAS is a critical component that carries vessels, nerves, and muscles of the nose. This layer extends from glabella up to the base of columella.[10] The dissection plan in rhinoplasty may be subcutaneous, sub-SMAS, or subperichondral.[11,12] Cakir and colleagues were the first who advocated subperichondrial dissection.[12] They demonstrated that this new approach can preserve all critical elements inside the SMAS

and provides a bloodless field intraoperatively and considerably reduces postoperative complications.[12]

Nasal ligaments and their clinical implications are the other emerging challenges in the applied anatomy of the nose.[23,24] Several definitive ligaments keep the stability of the nose and translate the functions of the nasal muscles to underlying structures. Destruction of the ligaments may affect both the aesthetic and functions of the nose.[24] Some investigators suggest the techniques to avoid these ligaments or to restore them by suturing back the ligaments to their place.[11,12,22] Main nasal tip ligaments are discussed in the following section.

Scroll Ligament

The scroll ligament is a longitudinal fibrous extension from the deep SMAS to the perichondrium of the scroll area (junction of the upper lateral and lower lateral cartilages) (**Fig. 4**).[23,24] Recently, it has been shown that transverse muscles of the

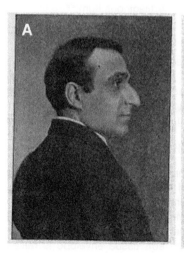
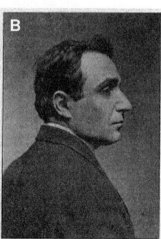

Fig. 3. (*A, B*) Lothrop's case for hump surgery. (*From* Lothrop OA. An operation for correcting the aquiline nasal deformity; the use of new instrument; report of a case. Boston Med Surg J. 1914;170:835–7.)

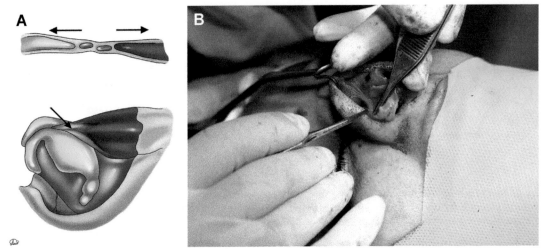

Fig. 4. (*A*, *B*) Scroll vertical ligament.

nose are attached to this ligament and elaborate their function on controlling nasal valves by this ligamentous attachment. This ligament can easily be damaged in cephalic trimming and as a result, the normal function of the nasal muscles will be disturbed or disabled.[24]

Interdomal Ligament

The interdomal ligament is a narrow strip of fibrous tissue that connects 2 dome segments at the cephalic portion of the cartilage.[23,24]

Intercrural Ligament (Suspensory Ligament)

Intercrural ligament (suspensory ligament) is a ligamentous connection between the cephalic border of entire alar cartilages. It holds to lower lateral cartilages together.

Pitanguy Midline Ligament

Ivo Pitanguy described a dermatocartilaginous ligament that originates from midline subcutaneous tissue and extends to domes and medial crura.[25,26] Later studies showed that the Pitanguy ligament is a fibrous extension of the medial SMAS that extends in 2 layers over and under the interdomal ligament. The upper segment is usually disrupted in open approach rhinoplasty. The lower branch extends to the membranous septum and attaches to the anterior nasal spin.[23,24] Some investigators believe that the Pitanguy ligament is critical in the stability of the nasal tip and need to be restored after tip plasty[12] (**Fig. 5**).

Pyriform Ligament

Pyriform ligament is a broad ligament that extends from nasal bones and pyriform aperture to both lower and upper lateral cartilage[27] (**Fig. 6**).

KEYSTONE AREA

Keystone is a bright word devoted by Cottle (1947)[17,18] to the region that 3 bony structures (2 nasal bones, the perpendicular plate of ethmoid) and 3 cartilaginous elements (2 upper lateral cartilages and nasal septum) unite.[13,28] As the name implies keystone works as the central stone in a gothic arch (osteocartilaginous vault of the nose) and when the central stone is removed (hump resection), reconstruction of this complex structure is not easy. Saban showed that keystone is a semimobile structure that by removing a strip from its underlying cartilage may move downward and eliminate the cartilaginous hum.[29]

BONY CAP

Palhazi and colleagues showed that bony hump is not the correct term. In fact, a thin bone layer covers a cartilaginous hump. They proposed a bony cap instead of the bony hump to show this anatomic finding.[13]

SURGICAL TECHNIQUES

Numerous techniques and modifications have been advocated for preservation hump surgeries that may seem very confusing and overwhelming.[29,30] Meanwhile, for simplicity, the whole process may be summarized in 4 consecutive steps. Firstly, the soft tissue envelope is raised

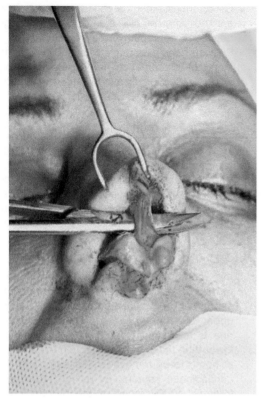

Fig. 5. Pitanguy ligament.

as a subperichondrial/periosteal flap. This may be done with limited dissections or wide approaches.[22,29] Then, a strip of septum is resected to created space for dorsal hump lowering.[14,22,24,29,30] The next step would be mobilizing the osteocartilaginous framework, which is done either as the push-down or as the let-down procedure. The last step would be stabilizing the mobilized dorsum in its new place.[29]

Soft Tissue Envelope Flap

Dorsal preservation techniques can be done both with open and closed approaches. The selection of the approach mostly depends on the complexity of the surgery and the surgeon's preferences. Dissections are done in subperichondrial/periosteal dissection plan to raise the envelope flap. This plan provides a bloodless field and causes minimal damage to nasal ligament.[11,12,22] Controversies in flap elevation may be summarized as follows:

- Open versus closed rhinoplasty: both may be applied based on preferences and complexity of the case and surgeon's preferences.
- Sub-SMAS versus subperichondrial plan: subperichondrial plan needs time to find the

plan, then it would less traumatic and more predictable.

- The extent of dissection: some surgeons prefer to avoid dissecting nasal ligaments as much as possible, whereas others prefer to have complete exposure and have a precise procedure especially when removing a bony wedge from the bony vault (let-down procedure). In wide dissections, ligaments need to be restored by precise suturing.

Mobilization of the Bony Vault

Push-down technique
When there is a small hump (less than 4 mm), mobilization of the bony vault is pushed down by push-down technique. In this technique, lateral and transverse osteotomies are done. Then the bony vault is mobilized and pressed done to its new position (see **Fig. 6**).

Osteotomies may be done by different modalities

- Saw: nasal saws are sometimes used to do the osteotomies.
- External 2-mm osteotome: lateral osteotomy is done as conventional to low osteopathy. A

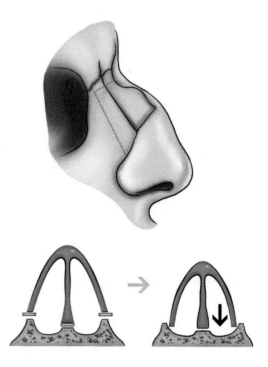

Push Down

Fig. 6. Push-down is performed by connecting lateral and radix transverse osteotomies and total mobilization of bony vault.

transverse radix osteotomy is added to make en bloc mobilization of the bony vault.

- Internal osteotomy: after performing lateral osteotomy, transverse radix osteotomy is added and the whole bony vault is mobilized in one piece.
- Piezosurgery: piezosurgery is a known instrument in rhinoplasty that provides a precise manipulation of bone and causes minimal damage to soft tissue. Nasal osteotomies by piezo is shown to be effective and safe.

Let-down technique

In the let-down technique, both lateral and transverse osteotomies are done. Then, a bony wedge is removed from the lateral wall of the bony vault to create the space for the downward movement of the bony vault.

In the let-down technique, in addition to lateral and transverse osteotomy, a wedge of bone is removed from nasofacial lateral wall (**Figs. 7** and **8**).

Bony wedge resection may be done with different instruments

- Bone forceps: Lathro[19] designed special forceps for bony wedge resection (see **Fig. 2**C). Although, regular bone rangeurs are frequently reported to be used for this purpose.

- Osteotomies: osteotomy lines are planned and marked. After precise osteotomy, the wedge between 2 osteopathy lines is removed.
- Piezosurgery: piezo has been used in different steps of preservation hump surgery. Bony wedge resection is a convenient indication for this technique.

Septal Strip Resection

A narrow strip of septum needs to be removed. Many methods have been advocated for septal strip. It is recommended that the septal strip be slightly wider than the excessive hump for better accommodation of the dorsum in the new position. The main methods for septal strip resection are as follows:

- Subdorsal resection (Saban's technique): in this method, 2 cartilage incisions are performed. The first one is in contact with the subdorsal vault (beneath the contact point of upper laterals and septum), and the second one is a straight incision a few millimeters lower than the first one (based on the amount of hump to be removed). After removing the cartilaginous septum, by using endoscopic forceps, small pieces of the perpendicular plate of the ethmoid bone are removed.
- High septal resection (Ishida, Most [modified high septal]): in this technique, cartilage

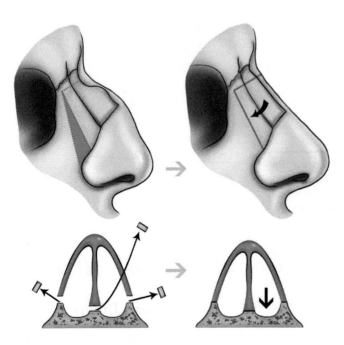

Fig. 7. In the let-down procedure, after performing all osteotomy, a bony wedge is resected from lateral nasal wall.

Let Down

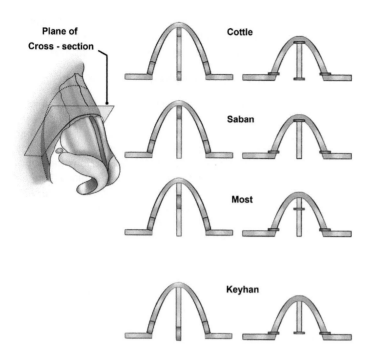

Plane of Cross - section

Cottle

Saban

Most

Keyhan

Fig. 8. Septal trip may be resected in different levels with different techniques.

incisions are made in the intermediate area of the cartilaginous septum, between subdorsal resection (Saban) and inferior resection (Cottle). In this method, 3 to 5 mm of subdorsal cartilage is left and 2 parallel incisions are done under the subdorsal cartilage. As originally described by most, in this technique 1.5 mm of the caudal septum may be left and 2 incisions are done behind this caudal strut.

Fixation and Stabilization

Recurrence of hump projection is an unman sequelae of the preservation surgery that may happen in 10% to 15% of cases. Fixation may considerably reduce the risk of recurrence. In high septal resections remnant of subdorsal cartilage is fixed to the nasal septum with several sutures. In subdorsal septal resections, these stabilizing sutures may be passed around the dorsum in septal angle and be fixed to the septum.

PRESERVATION HUMP SURGERY AND AIRWAY

In the early description, Goodale (1989) noticed that the nasal airway was not damaged in his case,[16] and later Lathrop (1914) was surprised that his patients felt better in nasal breathing.[19] There was no definitive reasoning for these findings till Saban hypothesized that upper lateral cartilages work as springs, and in preservative dorsal surgery, there is a vertical vector on nasal valves that by moving downward reinforces and improves the airway patency. On the other hand, in preservative techniques, nasal ligaments are left intact or precisely restored, which may be a determining factor in nasal airway function. Abdelwahab and colleagues[31] evaluated the effects of preservative and conventional hump surgery in a cadaver study and found that neither let-down technique nor conventional approaches reduced the internal nasal valve dimensions, although push-down reduced the internal valve area. Stergiou and colleagues[32] did the first clinical and radiographic study to assess the functional effects of dorsal preservation surgeries and found that these procedures considerably increase the internal nasal valve angle and improves nasal breathing. These initiative studies cannot provide strong evidence for a definitive conclusion. Meanwhile, it shows that preservative dorsal hump techniques are very promising regarding nasal functions.

PRESERVATION HUMP SURGERY NASAL AESTHETICS AND COMPLICATIONS

Several studies have evaluated safety, predictability, and aesthetic outcome of dorsal preserves surgeries. Saban and colleagues (2018) reported their long-term follow-up in a relatively large group of patients (320 cases). They stated successful results with a 3.4% revision rate (11 out of 320). In this case series, dorsal deviation, wide dorsum, and recurrence of the hump were the reasons for a few revision surgeries and no major complications such as saddle deformity and cerebrospinal fluid leakage were encountered. In Ishida's report (Ishida and colleagues,1998) (120 patients), both aesthetic and functional results were satisfactory and only 4 patients needed minor revision. In these series, recurrences of hump were seen in 15% of the patients. Almost similar results are reported by Saban and colleagues.[14]

That may show a relatively low risk of preservative techniques that are mostly very simple to be managed in revision surgery.

PRESERVATION RHINOPLASTY AND SIMULTANEOUS ORTHOGRAPHIC SURGERY

Rhinoplasty may be done as concomitant surgery with orthognathic procedures. Although the procedure is frequently reported in the literature. Many surgeons think that wide skeletonization in rhinoplasty will jeopardize the nasal framework and affect the safety of the surgery. Preservative rhinoplasty may solve many of these potential problems. Keyhan and colleagues showed how Le Fort I osteotomy may be comping to preservative hump surgery. In brief,

- Septal strip resection may be easily performed after a down fracture,
- Bony wedge resections and osteotomies can be performed with wider access and visibility, and
- Minimal dissections in rhinoplasty improve stability and predictability of the whole procedure.

LIMITATIONS OF PRESERVATION DORSAL HUMP SURGERIES

The outcome in preservative hump surgery directly depends on proper case selection, and preoperative analysis will be determinant. In many ethnic rhinoplasties such as asian and african noses, dorsal hump originates from tip under projection notthe defective dorsal structures. It is clear that structural rhinoplasty is the best treatment plan in these cases. Revision rhinoplasties are the other limitation in preservative techniques. In these patients, the internal nasal valve and keystone area may be damaged, and in many cases, there is no intact tissue to be preserved. Wide dorsum and deviated dorsum are 2 other relatively common rhinoplasty scenarios that need a direct approach to the cartilaginous vault. And sometimes spreader grafts and, on rare occasions, reduction and trimmings can easily solve the problems.

AUTHORS' COMMENTS

Preservative hump surgery has been opening a new era in rhinoplasty. The backbone of all preservative techniques is the recent anatomic findings and their practical applications. The nasal ligaments and their role in nasal functions cannot be underestimated. Subperichondrial dissection and preservations of ligaments as much as possible are 2 substantial rules in the preservation rhinoplasty. Meanwhile, there is no strict border between structural rhinoplasty and preservation rhinoplasty, meaning that even in structural rhinoplasty, it is feasible to apply these principles.

Keystone is the other anatomic element that is vastly studied. Now, it is clear that bony hump is not the proper name and bony cap is the best term that may show the anatomic details.

Current literature is completely supporting the safety of preservative hump surgery. It is claimed that preservative techniques may improve the nasal airway or at least does not damage it.

Limitations of preservative dorsal surgery are well understood, although it can be expected that future works will alleviate many of these shortcomings.

Finally, there is a growing challenge in selecting either preservative or structural rhinoplasty. It roughly reminds older debates in rhinoplasty on open versus closed approaches, and it seems that the same answer may arise very soon: "a rhinoplasty surgeon needs to be familiar with both preservative and structural rhinoplasty, master in one approach, and use the other in exclusive situations."

DISCLOSURE

The authors have nothing to disclose.

REFERENCES

1. Joseph J. Beiträge zur Rhinoplastik. Berl Klin Wochenschrift 1907;16:470–2.
2. Sheen JH. Aesthetic rhinoplasty. St Louis (MO): CV Mosby; 1978.
3. Sheen JH. Spreader graft: a method of reconstructing the roof of the middle nasal vault following rhinoplasty. Plast Reconstr Surg 1984;73:230239.
4. Bohluli B, Moharamnejad N, Bayat M. Dorsal hump surgery and lateral osteotomy. Oral Maxillofac Surg Clin North Am 2012;24(1):75–86.
5. Sharif-Askary B, Carlson AR, Van Noord MG, et al. Incidence of postoperative adverse events after

rhinoplasty: a systematic review. Plast Reconstr Surg 2020;145(3):669–84.

6. Lee M, Zwiebel S, Guyuron B. Frequency of the pre-operative flaws and commonly required maneuvers to correct them: a guide to reducing the revision rhinoplasty rate. Plast Reconstr Surg 2013;132(4): 769–76.

7. Byrd HS, Constantian MB, Guyuron B, et al. Revision rhinoplasty. Aesthet Surg J 2007;27(2):175–87.

8. B Bohluli, SC Bagheri. Chapter 104: revision rhinoplasty current therapy in oral and maxillofacial surgery.Saunders; 2012. p. 901-910.

9. Bohluli B. Esthetic rhinoplasty in the multiply operated nose. J Oral Maxillofac Surg 2019;77(7):1466.e1–13.

10. Saban Y, Andretto Amodeo C, Hammou JC, et al. An anatomical study of the nasal superficial musculoaponeurotic system: surgical applications in rhinoplasty. Arch Facial Plast Surg 2008;10(2):109–15.

11. Cerkes N. Concurrent elevation of the upper lateral cartilage perichondrium and nasal bone periosteum for management of dorsum: the perichondroperiosteal flap. Aesthet Surg J 2013;33(6):899–914.

12. Cakir B, Oreroglu AR, Dogan T, et al. A complete subperichondrial dissection technique for rhinoplasty with management of the nasal ligaments. Aesthet Surg J 2012;32(5):564–74.

13. Palhazi P, Daniel RK, Kosins AM. The osseocartilaginous vault of the nose: anatomy and surgical observations. Aesthet Surg J 2015;35(3):242–51.

14. Saban Y, Daniel RK, Polselli R, et al. Dorsal preservation: the push down technique reassessed. Aesthet Surg J 2018;38(2):117–31.

15. Daniel RK. The preservation rhinoplasty: a new rhinoplasty revolution. Aesthet Surg J 2018;38(02): 228–9.

16. Goodale JL. A new method for the operative correction of exaggerated roman nose. Boston Med Surg J 1899;140:112.

17. Cottle MH, Loring RM. Corrective surgery of the external nasal pyramid and the nasal septum for restoration of normal physiology. Ill Med J 1946;90: 119–35.

18. Cottle MH. Nasal roof repair and hump removal. AMA Arch Otolaryngol 1954;60(4):408–14.

19. Lothrop OA. An operation for correcting the aquiline nasal deformity; the use of new instrument; report of a case. Boston Med Surg J 1914;170:835–7.

20. Jammet P, Souyris F, Klersy F, et al. [The value of Cottle's technic for esthetic and functional correction of the nose]. Ann Chir Plast Esthet 1989;34(1): 38–41.

21. Ishida J, Ishida LC, Ishida LH, et al. Treatment of the nasal hump with preservation of the cartilaginous framework. Plast Reconstr Surg 1999;103(6): 1729–33.

22. Kosins AM, Daniel RK. Decision making in preservation rhinoplasty: A 100 case series with one-year follow-up. Aesthet Surg J 2020;40(1):34–48.

23. Daniel RK, Palhazi P. The nasal ligaments and tip support in rhinoplasty: an anatomical study. Aesthet Surg J 2018;38(4):357–68.

24. Saban Y. Rhinoplasty: lessons from "errors": From anatomy and experience to the concept of sequential primary rhinoplasty. HNO 2018;66(1):15–25.

25. Pitanguy I, Salgado F, Radwanski HN, et al. The surgical importance of the dermocartilaginous ligament of the nose. Plast Reconstr Surg 1995;95(5):790–4.

26. Pitanguy I. Revisiting the dermocartilaginous ligament. Plast Reconstr Surg 2001;107(1):264–6.

27. Rohrich RJ, Hoxworth RE, Thornton JF, et al. The pyriform ligament. Plast Reconstr Surg 2008;121(1): 277–81.

28. Irmak F, Ertaş A, Kaleci B, et al. The keystone, scroll complex, and interdomal area of the nose: histologic and anatomical observations. Plast Reconstr Surg 2020;146(1):75–9.

29. Patel PN, Abdelwahab M, Most SP. A review and modification of dorsal preservation rhinoplasty techniques. Facial Plast Surg Aesthet Med 2020;22(2): 71–9.

30. Lee J, Abdul-Hamed S, Kazei D, et al. The first descriptions of dorsal preservation rhinoplasty in the 19th and early- to mid-20th centuries and relevance today. Ear Nose Throat J 2020. https://doi.org/10.1177/0145561320925572.

31. Abdelwahab MA, Neves CA, Patel PN, et al. Impact of Dorsal Preservation Rhinoplasty Versus Dorsal Hump Resection on the Internal Nasal Valve: a Quantitative Radiological Study. Aesthetic Plast Surg 2020;44(3):879–87.

32. Stergiou G, Tremp M, Finocchi V, et al. Functional and Radiological Assessment After Preservation Rhinoplasty - A Clinical Study. In Vivo 2020;34(5): 2659–65.

Grafting in Modern Rhinoplasty

Steven Halepas, DMD[a], Kevin C. Lee, DDS, MD[a], Charles Castiglione, MD, MBA[b], Elie M. Ferneini, MD, DMD, MHS, MBA[c,d,e],*

KEYWORDS

- Rhinoplasty • Grafting materials • Rhinoplasty grafting techniques

KEY POINTS

- Grafts are applied for structural or cosmetic purposes to augment the existing nasal substructure. Stable clinical outcomes are achieved when the osseocartilaginous framework maintains its geometry and permits passive draping of the soft tissue.
- Autogenous cartilage, harvested as septal, costal, and auricular grafts, is the most biocompatible material.
- Commercially available grafts include processed homografts and synthetic implants. Although these can be obtained in abundant supply, they are known to cause long-term complications that are not seen with autogenous cartilage.
- Certain grafts are routinely used by all rhinoplasty surgeons, and these common configurations are discussed. To a certain extent, the choice of grafting technique depends on surgeon preference and experience.

INTRODUCTION

Rhinoplasty is the third most commonly performed invasive cosmetic surgical procedure behind breast augmentation and liposuction.[1] It is considered one of the most technically demanding cosmetic surgeries because of its limited access and complex 3-dimensional anatomy. Furthermore, even with adequate experience, many surgeons often have difficulty predicting and accounting for subtle long-term postoperative changes.

Embryologically, the developing nasal septum has 2 components that mirror the pattern of palatal development. The lesser anteroinferior segment of the septum arises as a continuation of the medial nasal processes after they fuse to form the primary palate. The remaining bulk of the nasal septum derives from the frontonasal process, which grows inferiorly to fuse with the palatal shelves of secondary palate and the anterior septum of the primary palate. The result is a complete separation of the right and left nasal chambers. Like other craniofacial structures, the nasal septum is composed of a neural crest core that can differentiate into a variety of skeletal and connective tissue precursors. The septum is completely cartilaginous at birth; however, beginning at birth and continuing through puberty, the bony septum undergoes endochondral ossification. This process shapes the vomer and the perpendicular plate of the ethmoid. The anterior septum persists as the quadrangular cartilage, which is a smooth, elastic hyaline cartilage that is composed of a type II

[a] Division of Oral & Maxillofacial Surgery, Columbia University Medical Center, New York-Presbyterian, 622 West 168th Street, Suite 7-250, New York, NY 10032, USA; [b] Division of Plastic Surgery, Hartford Hospital and Connecticut Children's Medical Center, University of Connecticut School of Medicine, 399 Farmington Avenue, Suite 210, Farmington, CT 06032, USA; [c] Beau Visage Med Spa, Cheshire, CT, USA; [d] Department of Surgery, Frank H Netter MD School of Medicine, Quinnipiac University, Hamden, CT, USA; [e] Division of Oral & Maxillofacial Surgery, University of Connecticut, Farmington, CT, USA
* Corresponding author. 435 Highland Avenue, Suite 100, Cheshire, CT 06410.
E-mail address: eferneini@yahoo.com

Oral Maxillofacial Surg Clin N Am 33 (2021) 61–69
https://doi.org/10.1016/j.coms.2020.09.003

collagen. Although cartilage is metabolically active, it is avascular and relies on diffusion to obtain adequate nutrition. Therefore, following injury, cartilage has a limited capacity for repair and regeneration. Grafting the nasal region with cartilage is a technical and biologic challenge because long-term graft survival is less reliable compared with skin and bone.[2]

Although the entire nose was originally considered a single unit of the face,[3] authors have long come to appreciate the complexities of functional and aesthetic nasal anatomy. Burget and Menick[4] first described the principles of nasal aesthetic subunits, which divided the external nose into a tip, dorsum, sidewalls, alar lobules, and soft tissue triangles. Other authors have since offered their modifications and even created separate classifications based on skin quality, light shadows, and underlying support. The nasal framework is best studied by dividing the nose into horizontal thirds. The upper third is supported by a bony vault, whereas the middle and lower thirds overlie a sophisticated cartilaginous substructure.[5]

Grafting is an essential component of primary and revision rhinoplasties and is performed for structural and/or cosmetic purposes. The reinforcement provided by structural or functional grafts permits the nose to resist static gravitational forces and dynamic forces that are applied during animation and respiration. There is tremendous variation in graft nomenclature, and this is often a source of confusion. Grafts are classified by their material, shape, number, location, or function. Furthermore, grafts are globally categorized as being either viable or nonviable. A nonviable graft has no direct contact to skin and is frequently used to provide structure. A viable graft has direct contact with the skin and is typically used for cosmetic purposes.[6] Unfortunately, the evidence supporting individual graft selection is limited. To a certain extent, the choice of graft for a given purpose is subject to provider preference and comfort. No randomized clinical trials have been conducted comparing graft materials and techniques for specific indications. Luckily, different grafts are deployed reliably with successful outcomes. In this review, we describe the most popular grafting materials and introduce common techniques used in the modern rhinoplasty.

GRAFTING MATERIALS

Whenever grafting is necessary, the septal cartilage is the preferred donor site because it is readily available and easy to access. When septal cartilage is unavailable or insufficient, acceptable autogenous alternatives include rib or concha.

Other sources of cartilage are available in rare circumstances. For example, during facial feminization surgery the use of cartilage from a concurrent thyroid chondroplasty has been described.[7] Secondary extranasal sources of grafting are more than twice as likely to be required with revision rhinoplasties.[8] Homografts and alloplastic biomaterials are available if autogenous donor sites are exhausted or undesirable. Each material described serves a purpose, but some materials are more versatile than others.

Septal Cartilage

Septal cartilage is widely accepted to be the best grafting material whenever it is available. The septum is always part of the surgical field, and septoplasty is often simultaneously planned for many patients. Septal cartilage is straight and resilient, and the biochemical composition is identical to that of the rest of the nose. Septal cartilage is less firm than costal cartilage, and some surgeons may prefer the later when a high value is placed on structural integrity. Graft size is the primary limiting factor, because a minimum 1 cm of septal cartilage needs to be preserved dorsally and caudally to serve as an L-shaped strut. The amount of available septal cartilage is subject to individual variability and is estimated with preoperative imaging. Postoperatively, septal perforation may require secondary surgical correction if the mucoperichondrial flaps are injured through and through.

Auricular Cartilage

The conchal bowl is accessed through either an antihelical or postauricular approach. The posterior approach has the benefit of a well-hidden incision, but proper technique results in inconspicuous scaring with either technique.[9] During harvest, care must be taken to preserve the antihelix and the crus helix, the latter of which divides the conchal bowl into the cymba and cavum. Conchal cartilage is generally thicker and more pliable than the septal cartilage. The entire segment possesses a curvature that may be advantageous for certain locations. The cymba concha is wider and thinner than the cavum concha.[10] Because of its 3-dimensional contour and resemblance, the concha is the optimal choice for lower lateral cartilage and alar reconstruction. The firmness, thickness, and concave shape of the cavum concha make it favorable for use as a shield graft. The intervening extension of the helical root is the most robust portion of the conchal graft, and as such it is used as a columellar strut.[11]

In the graft-depleted patient, the tragal cartilage graft is considered a salvage procedure. One cadaver study determined that the mean graft size that could be reliably harvested without visible deformities was 21.6 mm by 15.3 mm.[12] Those grafts were approximately 1 mm thick and similarly curved along the long axis. As with conchal cartilage, a stacked configuration or other modification is required to create a straight graft.

Costal Cartilage

The costal cartilage graft is the procedure of choice for total nasal reconstruction because of its volume and strength.[13] A tremendous amount of cartilage can be harvested from the rib's attachment to the sternum, and this abundance of material is sufficient to reconstruct even the most deficient dorsum. Costal cartilage has more than 4 times the average surface area of auricular cartilage,[9] and donor segments up to 5 cm in length are possible.[14] Exposure of the fifth or sixth rib is straightforward; however, the greatest care must be taken during dissection of the cartilaginous cap away from the underlying parietal pleura (**Fig. 1**). Whenever possible, the left ribs are preserved to avoid masking cardiac pain postoperatively.

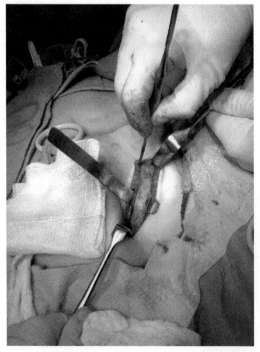

Fig. 1. Intraoperative dissection for harvesting a costal cartilage graft. Note the osseocartilaginous junction, which marks the lateral extent of available cartilage.

The disadvantages of harvesting costal cartilage include donor site morbidity, graft warping, and graft calcification. The donor site scar is typically well hidden. However, before closure, the wound should be filled with saline and examined for bubbling during Valsalva maneuver.[15] Chest tubes are not needed for most small pleural tears. Costal cartilage has an inherent and unpredictable tendency to warp over time, and this can cause residual deformity in the reconstructed nose. Strategies to reduce warping include increasing graft thickness,[16] performing balanced cross-sectional carving with central harvest,[17] including a chimeric osseous framework,[18] and using internal fixation with Kirschner wires or screw fixation.[19] Older patients have greater calcification of their costal cartilage. This calcified cartilage is less prone to deformation, but it is also more difficult to harvest and carve and is less predictably resorbed by the body.

Homograft Costal Cartilage

Nonautogenous grafts are composed of either synthetic or nonsynthetic materials, the latter of which include homografts. Irradiated homograft costal cartilage provides the option for structural grafting without the requirement of a separate donor site. These grafts are obtained from prescreened donor cadavers and subjected to 60,000 Gy of radiation. As with all donor tissue transfers, disease transmission is a theoretic possibility that is almost nonexistent in clinical practice. The primary concerns with irradiated homografts are the increased tendency to experience warping, resorption, and infection compared with autografts.[20] Resorption is particularly problematic because the graft is often applied as a load-bearing graft. Newer processing techniques have been described to overcome the limitations with irradiated grafts. Fresh frozen, nonirradiated costal cartilage is decontaminated using light surfactant to remove blood, lipid, and cellular components and antibiotic solution to remove donor pathogens.[21] Because there is no irradiation, this processing technique theoretically sterilizes the graft without affecting its viability. A recent study of 50 patients who underwent secondary rhinoplasty reported satisfactory outcomes without significant graft resorption.[21] The one case of infection that the authors encountered was treated effectively with light debridement and antibiotics.

Alloplastic Materials

The ideal facial implant is biocompatible, inert, becomes well integrated, and is easily contoured. Synthetic implants have many advantages including the lack of additional donor site, abundant supply, and the ability to be patient specific and maintain a reliable shape without concern for resorption. Commonly used alloplastic materials include silicone, porous high-density polyethylene (Medpor, Stryker, Kalamazoo, MI), and expanded polytetrafluoroethylene (Gore-Tex, W.L. Gore and Associates, Newark, DE). It is our opinion that the use of synthetic implants be restricted to immobile areas, such as the nasal dorsum. In general, alloplastic materials are often avoided in rhinoplasty because of safety concerns. It should be noted that silicone is still commonly used in Asian rhinoplasties because of its low cost, easy availability, and familiarity among providers and patients.

The physical characteristics of alloplastic implants determine their biologic behavior. Medpor, Gore-Tex, and silicone are all commercially available as sheets or preformed blocks. In addition, Medpor is thermoplastic and can be molded in situ to the desired shape and contour. Both Medpor and Gore-Tex are porous implants that allow for soft tissue ingrowth. Pores as narrow as 1 μm permit the translocation of bacteria, whereas macrophages require pore diameters of 30 to 50 μm. Because the pore size of Gore-Tex implants is between 10 and 30 μm, there is theoretically an increased risk of infection because of its semipermeability to bacteria. Medpor implants have pore sizes between 100 and 300 μm, and this feature is thought to reduce their incidence of infection.[22] Smooth, nonporous implants, such as silicone, rely on fibrous encapsulation for stabilization. All synthetic implants are prone to migration and extrusion; however, silicone implants seem to carry the greatest risk of both (**Fig. 2**). Implant retrieval rates have been estimated at 12%, 4.5%, 3.6%, and 2% for silicone,

Medpor, Gore-Tex, and combined materials, respectively.[23] As a general rule, oversized implants should be avoided, and recipient tissues should be thick, well vascularized, and closed with minimal tension.

GRAFT USE IN RHINOPLASTY

Grafts are performed for functional and/or aesthetic purposes. Grafting techniques are organized by their location.

Nasal Tip

Each lower lateral cartilage is divided into a medial, intermediate, and lateral crus. The medial crura contact the nasal septum, whereas the lateral crura follow curvilinear courses cephalically toward the piriform aperture. The intermediate crura lie between the medial and lateral crura, and its apex is the tip defining point.[24] The lower lateral cartilage connects to the upper lateral cartilage in a union that is referred to as the "scroll area."[25] According to the tripod theory, the nasal tip derives its support from the paired lower lateral cartilages. The 2 lateral crura each represent a leg of the tripod with the conjoined medial crura and caudal septum acting as the third leg. Maneuvers that increase or decrease the length these limbs in turn alter tip projection and rotation.[26]

The columellar strut graft is the workhorse graft for stabilizing the nasal tip (**Fig. 3**). For reference, a strut graft is a generic mechanical term describing any functional graft that provides outward-facing support. The columellar strut graft is placed between the medial crura and secured to the caudal septum (**Fig. 4**). Septal and costal cartilage are the preferred donor sites for the columellar strut because of their stiffness. Auricular cartilage is used when arranged as a double layer. When there

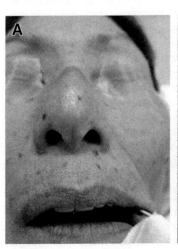 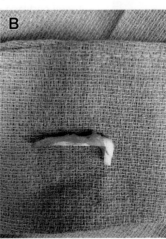

Fig. 2. Previously placed silicone implant that had migrated. The implant caused distortion of the soft tissue (*A*) and was subsequently removed (*B*).

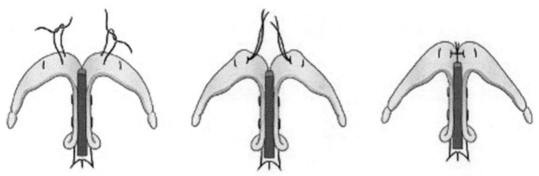

Fig. 3. The columella strut graft. Cartilage is placed between the medial crura and secured with sutures to provide increased tip support. (*From* Koehler JK. Basic rhinoplasty. In: Fonseca R, editor. Oral and maxillofacial surgery, volume 3. St. Louis: Elsevier; 2017. p. 374; with permission.)

is a lack of tip support, the columellar strut projects and restores the medial crural limb of the tripod. When existing tip support is adequate, the columellar strut may not be the most efficient means for just increasing nasal projection. To soften and augment the nasal tip, remnant cartilage is used to fill the open spaces and clefts at the nasal tip. If further projection is required, an onlay tip graft is placed in either a single or multilayered fashion over the alar domes. An onlay graft is a general term that describes any graft laid directly onto its recipient surface. These grafts can also mask tip asymmetries and should always be beveled along at the edges to blend with the surrounding cartilage. The onlay tip graft is termed a "peck graft" when it is applied in a transverse rectangular configuration. The combination of an onlay tip graft with a columellar strut is referred to as an "umbrella graft." Another onlay graft used to increase not only tip projection but also

rotation is the shield graft. This trapezoid-shaped graft sits anteriorly over the intermediate crura and travels inferiorly to the medial crural footplates.[27] In this position, it provides definition to the tip and supports the infratip lobule (**Fig. 5**). Extending the graft beyond the nasal dome provides additional projection, but this modification requires stabilization with a small interpositional block graft in the posterior dead space.

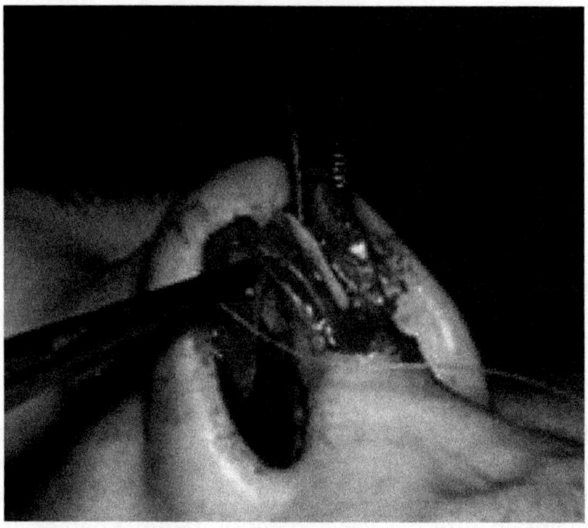

Nasal Dorsum and Septum

The spreader graft is a longitudinal graft that is placed often bilaterally between the dorsal septum and the upper lateral cartilages. Spreader grafts are considered the mainstay of treatment of internal valve collapse (**Fig. 6**). These grafts not only act as spacers to prevent narrowing of the internal valve angle, but they also widen and straighten the external appearance of the middle vault (**Fig. 7**).[24,28] They are often placed following dorsal hump reduction to close the open roof and reconstruct the disrupted internal valve. During the dissection, it is important to completely peel the mucosa off the deep aspect of the upper lateral process. Without adequate development of the submucoperichondrial pocket, graft placement may actually decrease apical angle and worsen internal valve obstruction.[29] Extended spreader grafts are designed to project caudally into the tip-lobule complex, and these longer grafts are combined with a columellar strut to recreate a composite L-shaped strut. Extended spreader can also be used with septal extension grafts to lengthen the nose. Septal extension grafts are straight grafts that are sutured end-to-end to the caudal edge of the septum. They directly lengthen the deficient septum and can project and derotate the nasal tip. Tip asymmetry is the main concern when using septal extension grafts, and care should be taken ensure a midline position during

Fig. 4. Columella strut graft placed for tip support. (*Courtesy of* Michael J. Will, MD, DDS, FACS, Will Surgical Arts, Ijamsville, MD.)

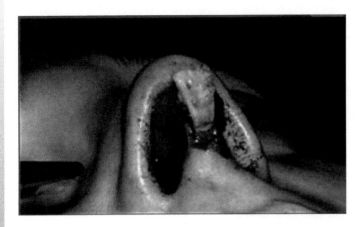

Fig. 5. Shield graft sutured in place. (*Courtesy of* Michael J. Will, MD, DDS, FACS, Will Surgical Arts, Ijamsville, MD.)

fixation. The butterfly graft was first introduced as an alternative to the spreader graft in revisional rhinoplasty but has gained popularity in addressing internal nasal valve compromise in primary and secondary cases.[30] It essentially functions like an external nasal dilator strip. The graft is usually shaped from conchal cartilage, placed superficial to the caudal septum, and sutured to the caudal margins of the underlying upper later cartilage.

Onlay grafts can also be placed over the upper lateral cartilages in the form of lateral sidewall onlay grafts. Like other onlay grafts, the purpose of these grafts is to mask uneven contours and irregularities. The dorsal onlay graft is another commonly used midvault onlay graft. They are often placed over the entire dorsal septum from the radix to the septal angle to reduce the risk of introducing additional irregularities. Whenever alloplastic materials or diced cartilage wraps are used, they are often used for this purpose. Diced grafts are useful when there is insufficient cartilage to harvest a single block graft, such as in the residual septum of a previously operated nose. They are placed either as a wrap or as free particulate. Diced cartilage grafts were originally described in 1942 but only gained popularity after 2000 following Erol's[31] publication describing his technique for wrapping them in Surgicel. Because of issues with graft resorption and foreign body reactions, Daniel and Calvert[32] modified the technique by wrapping their grafts in temporal fascia. Alternative protocols have since been described. Tasman and colleagues[33] impregnated diced cartilage with thrombin components of fibrin glue

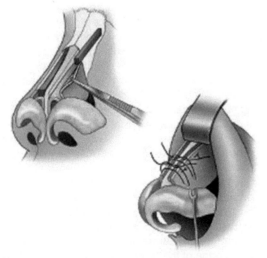

Fig. 6. Placement of a spreader graft between the nasal septum and upper lateral cartilages. (*From* Koehler JK. Basic rhinoplasty. In: Fonseca R, editor. Oral and maxillofacial surgery, volume 3. St. Louis: Elsevier; 2017. p. 371; with permission.)

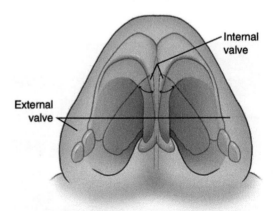

Fig. 7. Demonstration of the internal and external nasal valves. A minimum angle of 10° to 15° between the septum and upper lateral cartilage is needed to maintain internal valve patency. (*From* Koehler JK. Basic rhinoplasty. In: Fonseca R, editor. Oral and maxillofacial surgery, volume 3. St. Louis: Elsevier; 2017. p. 371; with permission.)

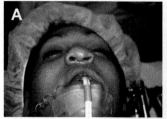
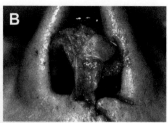
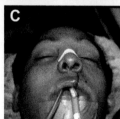

Fig. 8. Revision rhinoplasty for alar collapse in a patient born with cleft lip (*A*). Alar rim reconstructed with onlay graft (*B*). Immediate postoperative result (*C*).

(TISSEEL, Baxter International, Inc, Deerfield, IL). They found that their grafts were easier to manipulate into the desired shapes and sizes while demonstrating good long-term histologic viability and regeneration.[33] To limit inflammation and increase revascularization, Bullocks and colleagues[34] suggested the use of autologous tissue glue created from platelet-rich plasma. The preliminary outcomes with this approach are promising; however, the 1-year follow-up is too short of a period to adequately assess for resorption.

Alar Region

Alar rim contour grafts can correct or prevent alar retraction while simultaneously reinforcing the external nasal value. External valve collapse often results from overzealous resection of the lower lateral cartilages. In addition, alar notching is seen postoperatively when scar contracture deforms weakened lateral cartilages. Alar rim grafts are able to address both complications simultaneously.[35] The conventional rim graft is placed as a free-floating graft in a subcutaneous plane parallel to the existing or anticipated alar rim. The articulated modification involves securing the graft to the underlying tip. Composite alar grafts with skin and cartilage may be inserted to correct severe retraction and notching when there is insufficient soft tissue. The lateral crural strut graft is a more aggressive method for correcting alar rim deficiencies. This graft is placed as a supporting structure on undersurface of the lateral crus. By providing structural stability to the lower lateral cartilage, the lateral crural strut prevents alar rim collapse by tenting the adjacent soft tissue. From the basal view, this straightens out any lower lateral cartilage concavities and convexities. Unlike other lateral wall grafts, the lateral crural strut can also alter tip dynamics by repositioning the lateral legs of the nasal tripod. The alar batten graft is another graft that can fortify the nasal valves and increase their resistance to collapse. The alar batten graft is a curved rectangular graft that sits on the piriform rim laterally and overlaps the upper or lower lateral cartilage medially. An alar batten graft positioned caudally in the alar lobule can compensate for a deficient cartilaginous framework and correct alar retraction. When the graft is placed more cephalad, it can provide nasal sidewall support and reduce internal valve collapse. A final alar graft to consider is the lateral crural onlay graft. These grafts resemble alar batten grafts in that they rest on the surface of the lateral crus; however, like other onlay grafts they are designed to overlie and closely mirror the anatomy of the recipient surface (**Fig. 8**).

SUMMARY

Rhinoplasty is a highly challenging procedure that requires excellent surgical skills and extensive experience. The complexity is further emphasized by the countless number of grafting configurations that are possible. Postsurgical soft tissue changes are often dependent on the underlying bony and cartilaginous support in addition to the overlying skin thickness. Many rhinoplasty surgeons use workhorse grafts, such as the spreader graft and the columellar strut, to correct commonly encountered problems. Still, many grafting options exist, and there are many overlapping indications, such as when grafting the lateral wall. In those situations, rhinoplasty surgeons may have individual preferences based on their own comfort level and experiences. The authors have reviewed the main sources and configurations of rhinoplasty grafts. There is no substitute for high-volume experience, consistent practices, and the continued critical evaluation of functional and aesthetic outcomes.

CLINICS CARE POINTS

- Rhinoplasty is a highly challenging procedure that requires excellent surgical skills and experience.
- Autogenous cartilage remains the most biocompatible material.
- The septal cartilage is the preferred donor site because it is readily available and easy to access.
- Postsurgical soft tissue changes are dependent on the underlying bony and cartilaginous support as well as the overlying skin thickness.

DISCLOSURE

The authors have nothing to disclose.

REFERENCES

1. National plastic surgeon statistics. American Society of Plastic Surgeons; 2018. Available at: https://www.plasticsurgery.org/news/plastic-surgery-statistics?sub=2018+Plastic+Surgery+Statistics.
2. Grasso JA. Development of the head, face and mouth. In: Hand AR, Frank ME, editors. Fundamentals of oral histology and physiology. Hoboken: Wiley Blackwell; 2014.
3. Gonzalez-Ulloa M, Castillo A, Stevens E, et al. Preliminary study of the total restoration of the facial skin. Plast Reconstr Surg (1946) 1954;13(3):151–61.
4. Burget GC, Menick FJ. The subunit principle in nasal reconstruction. Plast Reconstr Surg 1985;76(2):239–47.
5. Joseph AW, Truesdale C, Baker SR. Reconstruction of the nose. Facial Plast Surg Clin North Am 2019;27(1):43–54.
6. Gunter JP, Rohrich RJ, Friedman RM. Classification and correction of alar-columellar discrepancies in rhinoplasty. Plast Reconstr Surg 1996;97(3):643–8.
7. Nesiba JR, Caplin C, Nuveen EJ. A contemporary and novel use of thyroid cartilage for structural grafting in esthetic rhinoplasty: a case report. J Oral Maxillofac Surg 2019;77(3):639.e1-7.
8. Lee LN, Quatela O, Bhattacharyya N. The epidemiology of autologous tissue grafting in primary and revision rhinoplasty. Laryngoscope 2019;129(7):1549–53.
9. Ho T-VT, Cochran T, Sykes KJ, et al. Costal and auricular cartilage grafts for nasal reconstruction: an anatomic analysis. Ann Otol Rhinol Laryngol 2017;126(10):706–11.
10. Mowlavi A, Pham S, Wilhelmi B, et al. Anatomical characteristics of the conchal cartilage with suggested clinical applications in rhinoplasty surgery. Aesthet Surg J 2010;30(4):522–6.
11. Boccieri A, Marano A. The conchal cartilage graft in nasal reconstruction. J Plast Reconstr Aesthet Surg 2007;60(2):188–94.
12. Rabie AN, Chang J, Ibrahim AM, et al. Use of tragal cartilage grafts in rhinoplasty: an anatomic study and review of the literature. Ear Nose Throat J 2015;94(4–5):E44–9.
13. Moretti A, Sciuto S. Rib grafts in septorhinoplasty. Acta Otorhinolaryngol Ital 2013;33:190–5.
14. Robotti E, Penna WB. Current practical concepts for using rib in secondary rhinoplasty. Facial Plast Surg 2019;35(1):31–46.
15. Cochran CS. Harvesting rib cartilage in primary and secondary rhinoplasty. Clin Plast Surg 2016;43(1):195–200.
16. Hakimi AA, Foulad A, Ganesh K, et al. Association between the thickness, width, initial curvature, and graft origin of costal cartilage and its warping characteristics. JAMA Facial Plast Surg 2019;21(3):262–3.
17. Gibson T, Davis WB. The distortion of autogenous cartilage grafts: its cause and prevention. Br J Plast Surg 1957;10:257–74.
18. Hsiao YC, Abdelrahman M, Chang CS, et al. Chimeric autologous costal cartilage graft to prevent warping. Plast Reconstr Surg 2014;133(6):768e–75e.
19. Gunter JP, Clark CP, Friedman RM. Internal stabilization of autogenous rib cartilage grafts in rhinoplasty: a barrier to cartilage warping. Plast Reconstr Surg 1997;100(1):161–9.
20. Wee JH, Mun SJ, Na WS, et al. Autologous vs irradiated homologous costal cartilage as graft material in rhinoplasty. JAMA Facial Plast Surg 2017;19(3):183–8.
21. Mohan R, Shanmuga Krishnan RR, Rohrich RJ. Role of fresh frozen cartilage in revision rhinoplasty. Plast Reconstr Surg 2019;144(3):614–22.
22. Ferneini E, Halepas S. Antibiotic prophylaxis in facial implant surgery: review of the current literature. Conn Med 2018;82(10):693–7.
23. Liang X, Wang K, Malay S, et al. A systematic review and meta-analysis of comparison between autologous costal cartilage and alloplastic materials in rhinoplasty. J Plast Reconstr Aesthet Surg 2018;71(8):1164–73.
24. Koehler J. Basic rhinoplasty. In: Fonseca R, editor. Oral and maxillofacial surgery, vol. 3, 3rd edition. New York: Elseiver; 2017.
25. Lam SM, Williams EF. Anatomic considerations in aesthetic rhinoplasty. Facial Plast Surg 2002;18(4):209–14.
26. Koehler J, Waite PD. Basic principles of rhinoplasty. In: Miloro M, Ghali G, Larsen P, et al, editors.

Peterson's principles of oral and maxillofacial surgery, vol. 2, 3rd edition. Shelton (CT): People's Medical Publishing House; 2012. p. 364–78.

27. Sheen JH. Achieving more nasal tip projection by the use of a small autogenous vomer or septal cartilage graft. A preliminary report. Plast Reconstr Surg 1975;56(1):35–40.

28. Fedok FG. Primary rhinoplasty. Facial Plast Surg Clin North Am 2016;24(3):323–35.

29. Seifman MA, Greensmith AL. Spreader graft placement: location, location, location. J Plast Reconstr Aesthet Surg 2018;71(3):448–9.

30. Howard BE, Madison Clark J. Evolution of the butterfly graft technique: 15-year review of 500 cases with expanding indications. Laryngoscope 2019;129(S1):S1–10.

31. Erol OO. The Turkish delight: a pliable graft for rhinoplasty. Plast Reconstr Surg 2000;105(6):2229–41.

32. Daniel RK, Calvert JW. Diced cartilage grafts in rhinoplasty surgery. Plast Reconstr Surg 2004;113(7):2156–71.

33. Tasman AJ, Diener PA, Litschel R. The diced cartilage glue graft for nasal augmentation. Morphometric evidence of longevity. JAMA Facial Plast Surg 2013;15(2):86–94.

34. Bullocks JM, Echo A, Guerra G, et al. A novel autologous scaffold for diced-cartilage grafts in dorsal augmentation rhinoplasty. Aesthet Plast Surg 2011;35(4):569–79.

35. Orlando GJ, Marquez E. Alar rim reconstruction with autologous graft cartilage: external approach. J Craniofac Surg 2019;30(3):868–70.

New Concepts in Nasal Tip Rhinoplasty

James D. Frame, CF, FRCS(Plast)*

KEYWORDS

• Rhinoplasty • Alar cartilage • Nasal valving • Liquid rhinoplasty • Open and closed rhinoplasty

KEY POINTS

- Medical nasal tip rhinoplasty can reduce the bulk of soft tissue either via superficial epidermolysis using abrasion, lasers or plasma, or via deep dermis using radiofrequency. Hyaluronic fillers have become a mainstay in managing tip asymmetry and contour defects.
- Understanding the anatomy of nasal superficial muscular aponeurotic system, distribution of fat within the nose tip, and sebaceous thickness of nasal tip skin gives a clearer understanding of expected outcomes and duration of postoperative swelling.
- Alar base wedge excisions are becoming more popular and avoid nasal flare, especially when reducing forward projection and narrowing the tip via an open approach.
- Nasal tip narrowing is done best using internasal and intranasal sutures rather than resection of alar cartilages. Soft tissue relocation may be necessary.
- Onlay cartilage tip grafts are advised only when necessary, and the skin is relatively thick to avoid spiking and visible displacement. Inlay grafts are preferable to support the nose tip, to fill in contour defects medially, and as spreaders in the treatment of valving.

In a majority of cases, tip rhinoplasty is included as an integral part within a general rhinoplasty and may involve profile augmentation or reduction and infracture. There are many cases where tip surgery alone can suffice to meet the patients' needs and less aggressive mobilization of the tissues is of benefit, but the best exposure always is through an open approach.

A closed approach is perfectly feasible provided that adequate exposure to the middle, medial, and lateral crura can be identified preoperatively. These patients tend to have flared nostrils and larger apertures.

Increasingly, the modern tip rhinoplasty surgeon includes the use of hyaluronic acid (HA) fillers (liquid rhinoplasty) in the armamentarium as a simple and rapid means of correcting grooves and asymmetries around the rim, lateral crus, alar dome, supratip, and medial crura. With an immediate visible result, little downtime, and with little risk, it gives the patient a chance to see if major surgery actually is necessary. The plane for HA injection and the plane of dissection must be understood, and these are explained herein. In a competitive market, the rhinoplasty surgeon has to offer all modalities of treatment.

SURGICAL ANATOMY

- The natural nose tip has an intricate anatomic architecture and shape specific to the individual and is composed of skin, fat, superficial muscular aponeurotic system (SMAS), muscle, cartilage, and mucosa. Essentially, the nose tip is a composite of all these connective and epithelial tissues that are mobile and free to glide over the lateral cartilages cranially and are pegged medially by the loose attachment of each alar cartilage adjacent to the caudal septum (**Figs. 1** and **2**).

The School of Medicine, Anglia Ruskin University, Chelmsford, Essex, UK
* Springfield Hospital, Lawn Lane, Springfield, Chelmsford CM1 7GU, UK.
E-mail address: j.frame@btinternet.com

Oral Maxillofacial Surg Clin N Am 33 (2021) 71–82
https://doi.org/10.1016/j.coms.2020.09.015
1042-3699/21/Crown Copyright © 2020 Published by Elsevier Inc. All rights reserved.

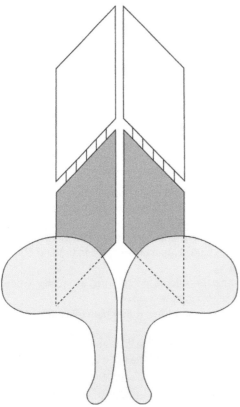

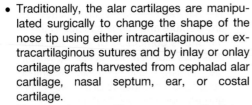

Fig. 1. Front-view drawing of nasal architecture showing overlap of the nasal tip alar cartilages over the lateral cartilages and implicating the relationship to nasal valving. The medial crus and foot process on each side is important in stabilizing the nose into a central position, but this centrality varies according to the axis of the septal cartilage. The arch of the middle alar crus, therefore, will be asymmetric if there is any septal angulation against which the medial crus is loosely attached.

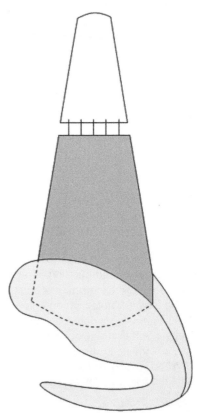

Fig. 2. Side-view drawing of nose showing overlap of the lower lateral cartilage by the lateral crura. To reduce the vertical height of the nose, the septum must be reduced in height and each of the lateral and medial crura also must be reduced in height. It is important to avoid intranasal soft tissue contracture by limiting unnecessary intranasal submucosal dissection of cartilages and to stabilize the nose tip against the septum at the time of surgery to prevent pollybeak deformity.

- Traditionally, the alar cartilages are manipulated surgically to change the shape of the nose tip using either intracartilaginous or extracartilaginous sutures and by inlay or onlay cartilage grafts harvested from cephalad alar cartilage, nasal septum, ear, or costal cartilage.
- There are loose and tenuous supporting intercartilaginous ligaments that suspend the alar cartilage composite from the underlapping lateral nasal cartilages and help maintain the nose tip gravitationally in a static position yet allow the nose to laterally flare or slide superiorly or inferiorly when animating and expressing.
- The lateral, middle, and medial crura of each alar cartilage spread the nasal os laterally to the left and right and are responsible for nasal

air entry and valving. The flexible external valve is influenced by voluntary movements of the small muscles attached to the lateral crus. These muscles are listed in **Box 1**. There is also splinting of alar soft tissues by accessory cartilage at the alar bases. The nasal tip can passively and voluntarily glide smoothly into a tip ptosis, or pollybeak, shape over the caudal midline cartilaginous septum but variable degrees of static ptosis of the tip often are hereditary and genetically predetermined. Postrhinoplasty swelling of the nasal tip is a cause of morbidity and can be explained by understanding the tissue plane of dissection in relation to the nasal SMAS.

- Accumulations of fat are present both superficial and deep to the alar SMAS layer,[1] and a complex of lymphatics, blood vessels, and

Box 1
Muscles acting on the nose tip and valves

- Levator nasii superioris alaeque nasi
- Alar nasalis
- Depressor septi
- Orbicularis oris
- Dilator naris anterior
- Compressor narium minor
- Transverse nasalis

nerves is transmitted in the more superficial layers with more solitary perforating larger vessels in the sub-SMAS layer of fat. This is relevant as a potential embolic danger when injecting fillers and assessing the potential for postoperative swelling and deep scar formation. There also is an interdomal fat pad and, where less developed, presents as a supratip depression in the diamond space above the medial alar domes.

- The plane and extent of tissue dissection required to expose and mobilize the alar cartilages during tip reshaping contribute to post-rhinoplasty tip swelling, which classically takes many months to settle. The thicker and more sebaceous the nasal skin (**Fig. 3**), the worse the postoperative edema within the fat pad and the longer time to settle, concomitant with patient disappointment if not adequately explained prior to surgery. These fat pads are not present over the upper lateral cartilages, and hence, there is less swelling postoperatively in these areas. The fat pads superficial to the SMAS at the nasal tip are also more spongy and vascular than in the sub-SMAS layer and contain diffuse cutaneous sensory nerve fibers to the tip. The larger individual sensory nerves and vessels travel in the sub-SMAS tissues before perforating into the superficial spongy layer through the loose interdomal and intercartilaginous ligaments.
- The fat compartments have no clearly defined borders and enable tissues to glide over a

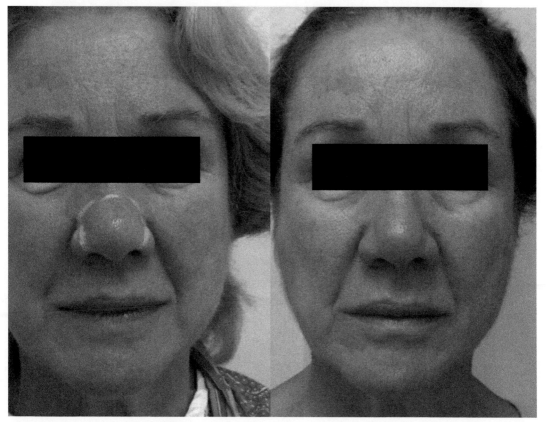

Fig. 3. Photograph to show thinning of thick sebaceous skin by superficial plasma energy treatment using Nebulaskin™ (manufactured by Fourth State Medicine). Left: Pretreatment. Right: Posttreatment with Nebulaskin™.

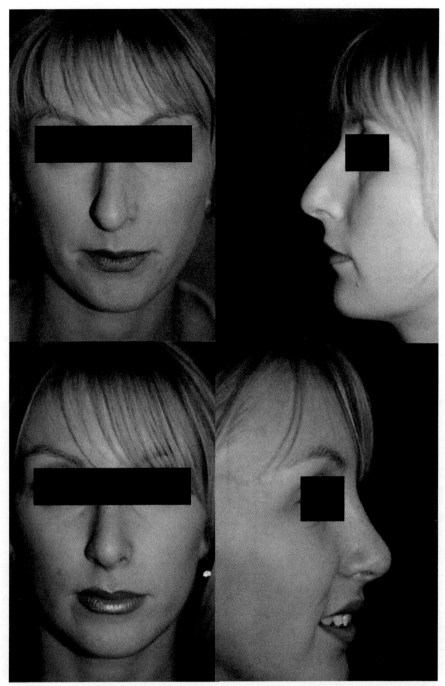

Fig. 4. A perceived attractive nose on front and profile views. Preperative views (upper left and right panels) and postoperative views (lower left and right panels).

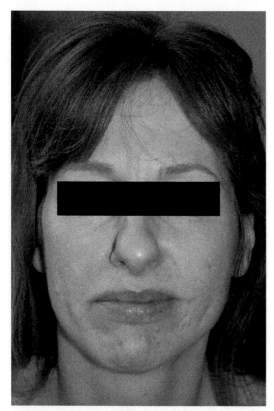

Fig. 5. Photograph of a box tip deformity.

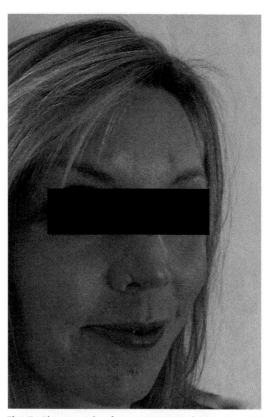

Fig. 7. Photograph of an overresected nose tip with excessive removal of basic structural support. The deeper dermal scar tightening means that the surface skin cannot be re-expanded.

fixed point and within the limits of muscle and fascial attachments. The function of SMAS is to position skin by attachment to the dermis via perpendicular structural ligaments and to transmit, distribute, and amplify the effect of contracting muscles by superficial containment. The more powerful the action the less compliant the SMAS layer.

- Steroid injections and therapeutic ultrasound may improve the duration of inflammatory edema in the fat adjacent to the SMAS but should be reserved for the patient with swelling associated with thicker sebaceous skin, to avoid thinning or depigmentation.

THE IDEAL NOSE TIP

In essence, the nose, however attractive, is one that is somewhat unseen when observed at first frontal facial glance, especially when great eyes, smile, lips, and white teeth are more the usual center of immediate attention (Fig. 4). High cheek bones and attractive nose are more obvious on profile view, but all assets are enhanced by hair color and hairstyle, skin quality, make-up, and

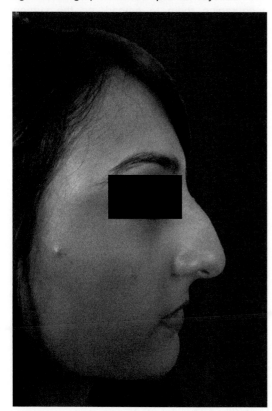

Fig. 6. Photograph of an ethnic nose and tip ptosis. In effect, there is a surplus of surface skin, and if the skin is sebaceous and spongy, there is limited improvement with tip rhinoplasty and a common cause of dissatisfaction to the patient.

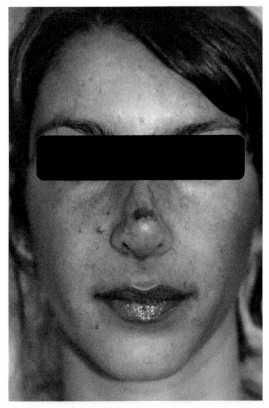

Fig. 8. Supratip ulcer after a fourth open rhinoplasty on a deeply scarred and immobile nose tip and use of aluminum nasal splint postoperatively attempting to reduce swelling.

clothes. The summation of all is beauty. There are many examples of high-profile attractive male and female celebrities who have attractive facial features yet ordinary noses.

The only person who is unhappy with the appearance of the nose nearly always is the person themself, and usually, it is a comment made in jest at a very young age at school that hurts and causes lasting concern to the patient, encouraging them to embark on the surgery route (**Fig. 5**). In men, skeletal prominence, facial skin texture, hairstyle, beard, and eyes tend to be the main features of attractiveness as long as the nose is not overly dominant on the face. In both sexes, the nose must be compatible but barely noticeable within the face. Most importantly, the nose tip must have the correct anatomic relationship to the remaining nasal skeleton and that suits the ethnicity of the individual (**Fig. 6**).

Box 3
Closed rhinoplasty limitations

Closed Tip Rhinoplasty: Procedures	Limitations
Alar cartilage mobilization and caudal trim	None. Easy release of alar chondromucosa
Alar cartilage riberration	None
Medial crus realignment	None. Limited exposure
Cartilage grafts—inlay/onlay	Reduced visibility with small/ptotic nasal os
Tip elevation and reshape	Reduced access in pollybeak or tip ptosis
Infill contour defects	Risk of graft displacement or malposition
Access to upper two-thirds nose	Positioning and stabilizing spreader grafts

---

Box 2
Approaches to the nasal tip

Closed Tip Rhinoplasty	Open Tip Rhinoplasty
• Intercartilaginous	• Extended rim incision transecting columella skin
• Intracartilaginous	• Low columella skin and midline tissue transection
• Rim incision extracartilaginous	
• Extended rim incision into columella	• High columella midline tissue transection

---

Box 4
Open rhinoplasty

Open Rhinoplasty	Limitations
Alar cartilage mobilization and caudal trim	None. Preservation alar chondromucosa
Alar cartilage riberration	None
Medial crus realignment	None
Cartilage grafts—inlay/onlay	None
Tip elevation and reshape	None
Infill contour defects	None
Access to upper two-thirds nose	None, especially for piezo osteotomy

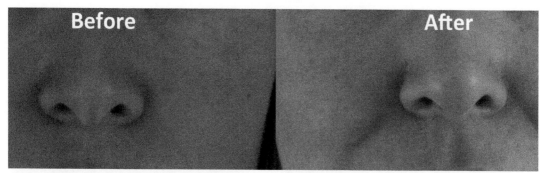

Fig. 9. Medial intercrural groove filled with HA.

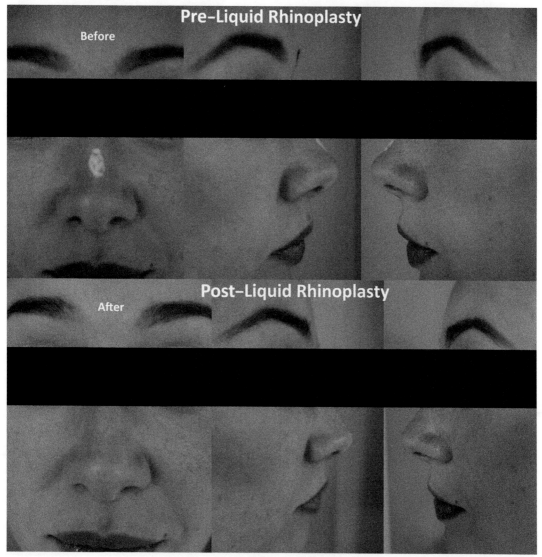

Fig. 10. Supratip and high nasal contour defects filled with HA to give the illusion of a straight nose.

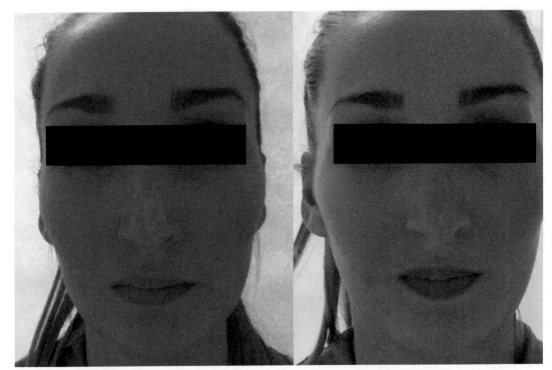

Fig. 11. Improvement of mild nasal valving using HA over the internal valve.

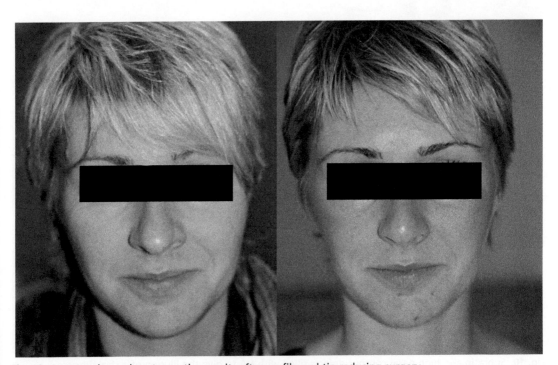

Fig. 12. Preoperative and postoperative results after profile and tip-reducing surgery.

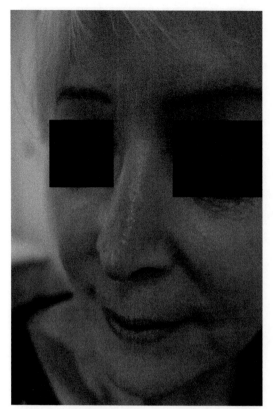

Fig. 13. A pinched nasal tip following excessive resection of alar cartilage.

Attractiveness is highly subjective of course and is perceived differently within and between ethnic groups. The importance of tip rhinoplasty is to avoid the overresected tip, often resulting multiple procedures in futile attempt to correct a heavily scarred and rigid tip with nubbins of remnant cartilage **Fig. 7**. The dangers of repeat open rhinoplasty attempting to improve nasal tip are relayed clearly in **Fig. 8**.

SURGICAL APPROACHES TO THE NOSE TIP

See **Boxes 2–4**.

LIQUID RHINOPLASTY

Supratip, intercrural, and nasal profile contour defects can be corrected easily using sub-SMAS HA (**Figs. 9** and **10**). Alar intranasal valving can be improved significantly with sub-SMAS HA filler (**Fig. 11**).

CLOSED TIP RHINOPLASTY

- A gentle manipulation and repositioning of the alar cartilages through a closed intercartilaginous approach can give an excellent tip appearance (**Fig. 12**). The patient who benefits is looking for minimal change and generally is happy with the original tip shape. A narrow tight tip with a nubbins look results if excessive resection is carried out (**Fig. 13**). The same result can be achieved by overtightening any intercrural or intracrural alar sutures. This risk of a pinched look is discussed best with the patient prior to surgery because less is nearly always better than more in alar tip surgery and sometimes compromise is needed. Although the intracartilaginous and rim incisions are useful in certain types of nose, they are less useful approaches if dorsal nasal work also is being performed, and there also is more risk of notching and rim retraction.
- Access for major tip suturing techniques using the closed approach is limited, especially when the nares are small or the tip is pollybeak. The box tip nose can be improved gently using the closed intercartilaginous approach with both surfaces of each alar cartilage dissected free of attachment

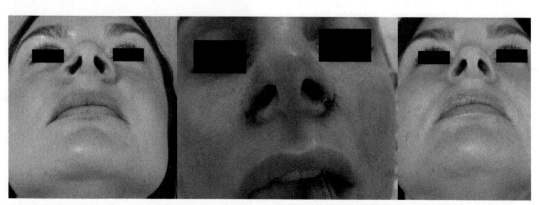

Fig. 14. Classical box tip nose deformity corrected by intra alar cartilage sutures and alar base wedge excisions. Preoperative view (*left*), perioperative view (*middle*), and postoperative view (*right*).

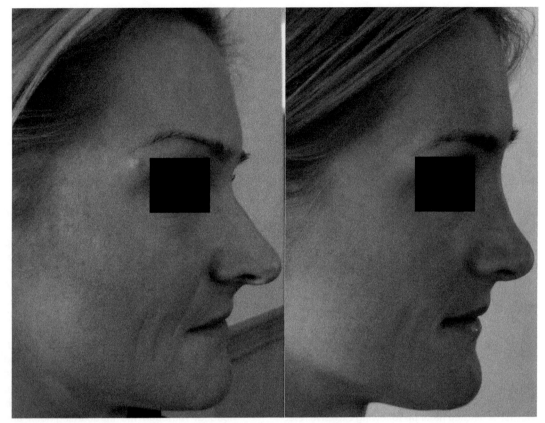

Fig. 15. Preoperative and postoperative lateral nasal views of a patient that underwent the Eiffel Tower procedure to reduce the projection of the whole nose, including tip complex.

(**Fig. 14**). Intracrural or intercrural sutures are eminently possible, because usually there is excellent exposure, especially if the incision is carried down into the columella. Through the same approach, the tip profile can be reduced by trimming cartilage segments off each medial and lateral crus—sometimes referred to as the Eiffel Tower procedure in Europe. Reducing the inevitable lateral alar flare intranasally but more often via an external resection of alar base both narrows and helps drop the vertical height of the nose (**Fig. 15**).

- Fixating the tip complex to the septum after disruption of the SMAS during elevation of the tissues is mandatory, either with sutures, inlay graft, or vertical strut graft. An interesting tip is to create a small notch on the low anterior dorsal septum to anchor the tip complex and prevent pollybeak or ptosis. This is known as the Hackett notch, as practiced by plastic surgeon Mike Hackett in the United Kingdom in the 1980s.

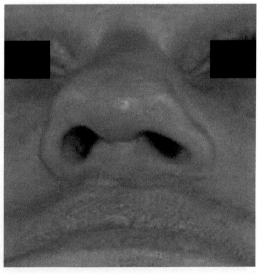

Fig. 16. The classic deformity seen when there is inexact closure of columella after open rhinoplasty.

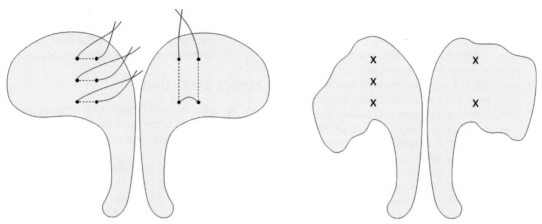

Fig. 17. Intracartilage suture techniques shown diagrammatically. The intention is to tighten the sutures and narrow the tip by making a more acute angle and without performing any riberration.

OPEN TIP RHINOPLASTY

Understanding the modern philosophy and the approaches now being made to primary rhinoplasty cannot be better described than within John Tebbetts' book.[2] The contemporary generation of plastic surgeons generally has been trained in the open approach yet there still are solid reasons for selecting a closed approach, especially where minimal tip work only is required.

- For accuracy of placement of sutures and grafts and alignment of tissues around the nasal tip, the open approach undoubtedly offers the best exposure, yet experienced surgeons can adapt and have now modified their open technique to the closed approach, where appropriate, to deliver the same outcome using the same intracrural and intercrural suturing techniques with or without cartilage grafts (Pshenisnov K, MD, personal

communication, 2018).[2] Good exposure to the tip and dorsum via an open approach, however, is essential if the modern concept of raising perichondroperiosteal flaps to be replaced after modifying the nasal profile, including the accurate placement and fixation of inlay and onlay grafts.[3,4] An open approach almost is mandatory for major secondary tip surgery involving cartilage reconstruction.

- The marginal incision in open rhinoplasty is placed adjacent to the mucosal rim of alar cartilage and extended over the middle crus into the columella. The transverse columella incision can be placed high or low, and it should be either stepped or chevron shaped but always carefully preserving the alar rim cartilage and the blood supply to the soft tissues within the flap. An exact anatomic closure is essential to prevent the classic deformities (**Fig. 16**). It is safer to elevate the

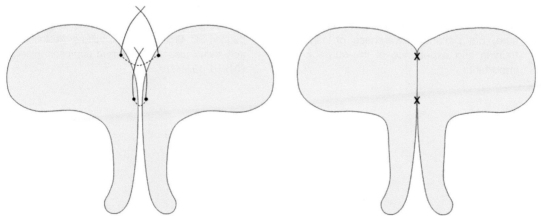

Fig. 18. Intercartilage suture technique to show how the nose tip can be elevated. Inlay grafts can be inserted between the medial crura to strengthen the support if suturing to the septum alone is inadequate.

tip through a transverse incision just anterior to the narrowest point of the columella if no medial crural work is required.

- Harvesting a cephalad strip of alar dome cartilage is useful in the event that tip grafts are required, but this must be kept to a minimum and great care must be taken to allow for mucosal retraction and inevitable fullness as the tip complex realigns with scar after the disruption of the nasal SMAS layer. This swelling takes at least 1 year to settle, and excessive excision can contribute to lateral wall collapse and valving, especially with concomitant nasal bone infracture. The less cartilage taken, the less dissection is required and the least morbidity. Removing lateral alar cartilage, especially for use as a graft, is advised only when reducing the anterior projection of nose and considering alar base reduction to prevent flaring. Excessive removal of this portion of lateral alar cartilage can cause a collapse and unsightly soft tissue groove on the rim.
- Intracartilage and intercartilage suture placements and intended outcomes are shown diagrammatically in **Figs. 17** and **18**.

SUMMARY

- The nasal tip is a complex composite of layered tissues that respond differently to trauma in each individual.
- Postoperative swelling of the nose tip takes at least 1 year but nearer to 2 years to settle.
- Liquid rhinoplasty can give excellent immediate and long-lasting results with minimal risk and little downtime.
- A closed tip rhinoplasty can offer acceptable results within the limitations of exposure for intradomal and transdomal cartilage suture and graft techniques.
- An open tip rhinoplasty gives the best exposure, but patient's awareness of risk and training and experience of the surgeon are important.

- Lesser resection always is better than over-resection of alar cartilage.
- The best chance of getting the best outcome for the patient is always at the first procedure.

CLINICS CARE POINTS

- Be sure to understand what change in the appearance of the nose the patient is seeking.
- Be sure that you can deliver the nose that is requested.
- Be prepared to manage the difficult patient.
- Be prepared to perform secondary surgery.
- It is wise to wait at least 1 year between primary and secondary rhinoplasty. Using fillers to fill contour defects can delay and obfuscate any need for surgery until the overlying tissues have softened.
- Try to avoid the horizontal columella incision in open rhinoplasty by extending the medial longitudinal incisions to relax tissues and provide adequate exposure to the dorsum and tip.

DISCLOSURE

The author has nothing to disclose.

REFERENCES

1. Saban Y, Andretto A, Hammou JC, et al. An anatomical study of the nasal superficial, musculoaponeurotic system: surgical applications in rhinoplasty. Arch Facial Plast Surg 2008;10(2):109–15.
2. Tebbetts JB. Primary rhinoplasty. A new approach to the logic and the techniques. Mosby; 1998. ISBN 0-8151-8892-7.
3. Pshenisnov K. Aesthetic nasal tip surgery. In: Frame JD, Bagheri SC, Smith DJ, et al, editors. Aesthetic surgery techniques. A case based approach. Elsevier; 2019. p. 121–32. ISBN:978-0-323-41745-7.
4. Cerkes N. The Middle-Eastern Nose. In: Frame JD, Bagheri SC, Smith DJ, et al, editors. Aesthetic surgery techniques. A case based approach. Elsevier; 2019. p. 137–46.

Rhinoplasty with Fillers and Fat Grafting

Mohammad Bayat, DDS[a,*], Naghmeh Bahrami, DDS, PhD[b,c], Hassan Mesgari, DDS[d]

KEYWORDS

• Rhinoplasty • Nonsurgical • Fat injection • Filler • Minor nasal deformity

KEY POINTS

• The use of fillers and fat graft is used only in cases of mild deformities and it should not be thought that this method can be an alternative to complete rhinoplasty in cases with definite indication.
• It is very important to pay attention to the microvasculature of the nasal area in injections because if the injection goes into the vessels, it can cause catastrophic events such as blindness or brain damage.
• Fat injection is a priority over fillers because it provides a larger volume of material and reduces the risk of unintended safety reactions. It is also unlikely to transmit disease. With new technology, it is possible to add cells and use tissue engineering in the fat graft technique, which gives a better chance of success.

INTRODUCTION

Today, the number of patients who desire to aesthetically improve the appearance of their nose without having to undergo surgical rhinoplasty has increased. Although surgical rhinoplasty is typically the choice of patients seeking aesthetic improvement of the nasal shape, using an injectable material for fixing irregularities and asymmetries holds great appeal owing to the simplicity of the correction, use of local or no anesthesia, comparatively low cost, and lack of downtime. In the majority of treatments, permanent or semipermanent fillers are injected into the dorsum, tip, and columella.[1]

A noninvasive method for nasal recontouring is to bypass permanent surgical correction, although these modalities are mostly impermanent.[2] In certain cases, secondary rhinoplasty can be an alternative; however, it can be laborious to perform, particularly if the skin is thin.[2] Moreover, the majority of patients decline to undergo a new procedure.[3,4]

There are various surgical and nonsurgical procedures for rhinoplasty. Augmentation can be performed by surgery and multiple graftings, such as cartilage or facial augmentation, permanent implants such as Medpore, poly(methyl methacrylate), silicone, and other materials. Nonsurgical rhinoplasty can also be carried out by injecting fillers (permanent, semipermanent, or resorbable) and with autologous fat transfer. Each procedure has its own advantages and disadvantages.

Numerous techniques have already been used to improve noticeable contour deformities and sharp edges of bone and cartilage to obtain a dorsum with a smoother contour and pad, especially for patients with thin dorsal nasal skin.[5–7] Autologous and alloplastic materials can cover the underlying osseocartilaginous framework. Temporalis fascia graft,[5,8] dermal fat graft,[5,8] Erol's diced cartilage graft,[9] and homografts such as acellular dermis (Alloderm; LifeCell,

[a] Department of Oral & Maxillofacial Surgery, Shariati Hospital, Tehran University of Medical Sciences, north kargar ave, Tehran Iran; [b] Department of Tissue Engineering and Applied Cell Sciences, School of Advanced Technologies in Medicine, Tehran University of Medical Sciences, north kargar ave, Tehran Iran; [c] Craniomaxillofacial Research Center, Tehran University of Medical Sciences, Tehran, Iran; [d] Facial Esthetic Surgery, Tehran University of Medical Sciences, north kargar ave, Tehran Iran
* Corresponding author. #1 no 28 Tir st Mahmudieh Avenue, Tehran 1986655355, Islamic Republic of Iran.
E-mail address: mobayat2000@yahoo.com

Oral Maxillofacial Surg Clin N Am 33 (2021) 83–110
https://doi.org/10.1016/j.coms.2020.09.004

Branchburg, NJ) are autologous materials that sporadically resorb and lose their ability as a camouflage.[7,10–12] Alloplastic materials such as polytetrafluoroethylene have a high incidence of infection.[13,14]

In rhinoplasty, both autologous grafts and synthetic implants have shown satisfactory outcomes. Synthetic implants, nonetheless, are associated with 2 major complications: displacement and extrusion.[15] With regard to these disadvantages, autologous cartilage and bone grafts are the choice of most patients owing to the excellent biocompatibility and low risk of infection and extrusion.[16] However, inconsistent volume and uncontrollable shape of the graft, an unreliable absorption rate, and possible donor site morbidity are disadvantages of autologous grafting.[16] A meta-analysis reported a number of complications after the implantation of alloplastic materials in rhinoplasty but supported the placement of alloplastic implants in case of unavailability or insufficiency of autogenous materials.[17] At present, there are no established guidelines for transplanting alloplastic materials.[18] The nonsurgical treatment of rhinoplasty sequelae was performed in 1904 by Stein, who injected paraffin to correct a saddle nose deformity[3,19]

INDICATIONS FOR NONSURGICAL RHINOPLASTY

Nonsurgical rhinoplasty, known as liquid rhinoplasty, is a general term for the correction of nasal defects. In fact, it is a nonsurgical procedure for corrective treatment of specific nasal areas, including saddle nose, contour deformities, side wall irregularities, hump removal, columella retraction, nasal lengthening, dorsal augmentation, deep radix, nasal tip projection and rotation, nasolabial angle, and asymmetry.[2]

The most common indications for fat injection (or autologous fat transplantation) after rhinoplasty include revision of dorsal, inverted V, stairstep, and saddle nose deformities.[20] In nasal scarring and tight thin skin, fat grafts are useful. Autologous fat grafts are thought to create a space between densely adherent skin and the underlying nasal skeleton, helping to camouflage deformities and making secondary procedures and subsequent dissection significantly easier.[1,20] The forehead–glabella–radix complex is another area where injecting fillers or fat and represents an essential triad in rhinoplasty, from which the nasofrontal angle is derived.[21] The radix is a depression at the origin of the nose,[22] and the nasion, or the bridge of the nose, is the depressed part of the nose, and is located 4 mm to 6 mm deep to the glabella, just below the eyebrows.[21] The nasofrontal angle is the transition between the forehead and the dorsum of the nose and can vary from 128° to 140°. However, the ideal angle for women is 134° and for men is 130°.[22]

Fat grafting to the radix may diminish complications of radix augmentation (visibility, resorption, and donor site issues); however, this method provides an easily available solution to the thick nasal base. Increasing the height of nasal radix minimizes the necessary amount for hump or tip modification.[23] This issue is very important in patients with thick nasal skin.[24] Cranial and caudal radix positions provide a longer nasal dorsum with a decreased anterior projection and a shorter nasal dorsum with increased anterior projection, respectively.[25] In addition, a deep and high radix decreases and enlarges the nasofrontal angle, respectively. Variations come with normal aging, especially those influencing bone, muscle, fat, and skin, and are determining factors of the nasofrontal angle. Age also causes the retrusion of the glabella and nasion.[26] Depression in the lower forehead and bossing of the forehead may be present owing to soft tissue atrophy or bony remodeling and hyperinflation of the frontal sinus, respectively.[27] A piriform aperture is an indicator for determining the nasolabial angle.[21] Midface retrusion mainly occurs with aging.[28] This aging process includes the piriform aperture, which remodels posteriorly relative to the upper face, resulting in a loss of bony support for the alar base.[12] In addition to piriform aperture, the anterior–posterior position of the alar base is another criterion affecting the nasolabial angle, which changes with age (**Fig. 1**).[21]

CONTRAINDICATIONS

Despite many benefits, injecting fillers or fat grafts to the nose has some limitations and contraindications. Nose injection is an augmentation procedure. Hence, an overprojected nose is not an indication for augmentation.[29] Injection of fillers is typically associated with local and systemic contraindications. An infected area, active viral infections like herpes, necrosis of the skin owing to prior interventions, and pimples are examples of local contradictions. Vasoconstrictors, which are commonly used in local anesthesia, are not appropriate for heavy smokers or patients with cardiovascular diseases.[30]

NASAL ANATOMY AND DANGER ZONES

The arterial supply of the nose is provided by branches of carotid arteries, namely, the

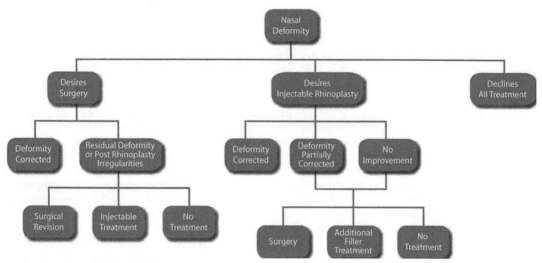

Fig. 1. Treatment algorithm for development of patient care treatment plan.

ophthalmic and facial arteries. The ophthalmic artery is derived from the internal carotid artery, the same as the vessels that come from the cavernous sinus. The central retinal artery is the first intraorbital branch and one of the most important and smaller branches of the ophthalmic artery. The ophthalmic artery has 2 terminal branches: the supratrochlear artery and the dorsal nasal artery. The dorsal nasal artery originates from the orbit above the medial palpebral ligament is divided into 2 main branches. The first passes through the root of the nose, and the second passes along the dorsum of the nose, which supplies its external surface area in its path toward the nasal tip. In addition, the first branch inosculates with the angular artery, whereas the second branch inosculates with both its fellow artery of the other side and the lateral nasal artery, which emanates from the facial artery and ascends along the side of the nose. The lateral nasal artery supplies not only the ala of the nose, but also the dorsum of the nose and inosculates with its fellow and the following branches: the septal and alar branches, the dorsal nasal branch of the ophthalmic artery, and the infraorbital branch of the internal maxillary. The columellar artery is the superior labial branch of the facial artery that runs up the columella, ends, and inosculates in the tip with the lateral nasal branch of facial artery.

The following are the major conclusions achieved from this anatomic review. There is a direct and short connection between the proximal blood supply of the nose and the internal carotid and retinal arteries. During injection in the area of the dorsum, radix, or glabella, this network can be affected by embolization and can cause various calamitous outcomes such as blindness or brain infraction. Embolization of the distal blood supply, which is mostly at the tip and in alar regions, also can give rise to a wide variety of ischemic phenomena.[2]

The cutaneous microvasculature in human skin is organized into 2 horizontally aligned plexuses that include 3 blood vessel segments: arterioles, venules, and the interposed arterial and venous capillaries.[31] Capillary loops are divided into 6 to 8 loops and extend into elongated the dermal papillae, which come directly from the perforating arteries of subcutaneous fat. In this structure, arterioles and venules are directly linked to the upper branchial plexus, where the majority of microvasculature is situated 1 to 2 μm below the epidermal surface. The arteriolar vessels in the papillary dermis vary from 17 to 22 μm in outer diameter, first decreasing to capillaries and then increasing to postcapillary venules (with the diameters from 4 to 6 μm and from 10 to 15 μm, respectively).[32–35] Many years ago, physiologists came to the conclusion that the skin's extensive blood supply is beyond its nutritional requirements and postulated that this structure serves to aid in controlling control body temperature.

Postcapillary venules are the largest part of vessels within the papillary dermis and represent the place where inflammatory cells move from the intravascular to the interstitial space and where acute inflammation occurs.[31,36]

The structure of the 2 layers of blood vessel is that the superficial plexus supplied by the vessels from the hypodermis include small conical areas at the center of the vessels feeding from the lower plexus.[37,38] Based on the 2-dimensional representation from the surface, the disks forming the borders of each cone create a pattern that is observable during vascular obstruction. This apparent pattern of a disk placed on the surface delineates these conical drainage areas from the superficial plexus to the deep one. For instance, livedo reticularis or mottled skin, which is a vascular reaction pattern, can frequently be observed in cases of skin thromboembolism. The main reason for this pattern is due to the slow flow of blood within the postcapillary venules.[38] Thus, the clinical pattern is related to blood stagnation in the dermal venules, and the bluish discoloration of the skin arises from desaturated blood, optically filtered by the dermis and epidermis (**Figs. 2** and **3**).[36]

FAT

The use of fat grafts for the correction of congenital malformations and intricate traumatic wounds

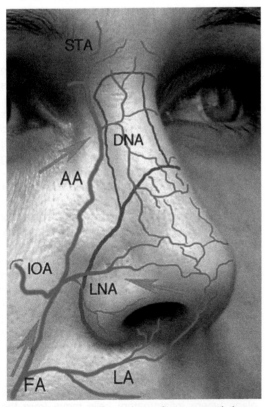

Fig. 2. Main arterial supply to the nose and danger zones regarding fat injection (*arrows*). AA, angular artery; DNA, dorsal nasal artery; FA, facial artery; IOA, infraorbital artery; LA, superior labial artery; LNA, lateral nasal artery; STA, supratrochlear artery. (*From* Monreal J. Fat grafting to the nose: personal experience with 36 patients. Aesthetic Plast Surg. 2011;35(5):916; with permission.)

with soft-tissue loss following radical surgery of tumor was proposed for the first time in 1893 by Neuber. This notion was followed by Hollander in 1912, by Neuhof in 1921, and by Josef in 1931[39] (**Table 1**). Liposuction and tumescent anesthesia were other techniques introduced by Fisher in 1974 and by Klein in 1985.[39,40] In 1919, Bruning used fat injection to correct postoperative cosmetic nasal deformities.[41] However, the technique was not sufficiently accepted owing to the poor survival duration of the fat grafts.[42,43]

Fat grafting continues to be one of the most common procedures because of the simplicity of fat harvest, the availability of graft materials, and the lack of transplant rejection. Nonetheless, the rates of fat survival and retention cannot be predicted, and various difficulties (eg, abscesses, cysts, nodulation, and neurovascular injury) may arise.[44] Later, after extensive research and improvement of surgical methods, structural fat grafting was recognized as a reliable treatment strategy with satisfactory clinical consequences.[45] In 2007, the idea of microautologous fat transplantation (MAFT) was presented by Lin and colleagues,[46] who suggested that this technique provides reliable results and is feasible in facial rejuvenation[18,47–51]

Because of its abundance, easy accessibility, lower cost, host compatibility, and repeated harvesting, fat has the potential for becoming the perfect soft tissue filler. Additionally, in comparison with dermal fillers, fat provides similar long-lasting durability with a low cost.[52,53]

Previous investigations have reported a broad variety of indications for fat grafting, including cosmetic improvement, body contouring, scar reconstruction, periocular rejuvenation, progressive hemifacial atrophy, radiation-damaged sites, and fat atrophy in patients infected with the human immunodeficiency virus. In this field, much progress has been achieved; however, tumescence of the base of all these fat graft surgeries is tumescence anesthesia.[54]

In 2009, fat grafting constituted 5.9% of all nonsurgical cosmetic procedures.[55] This technique has widely been applied in the rejuvenation of different parts of the body, the correction of deformities caused by liposuction, and aesthetic refinement of body contours such as the buttocks.[56] The method of fat injection into the nose helps to cover deficiency of a former rhinoplasty or enhance skin thickness in cases with a skeletonized nose[57] or in cases involving congenital, posttraumatic, or traumatic pituitary soft tissue defects.[14] Facial rejuvenation and contour enhancement using fat grafting, as a filler, has shown

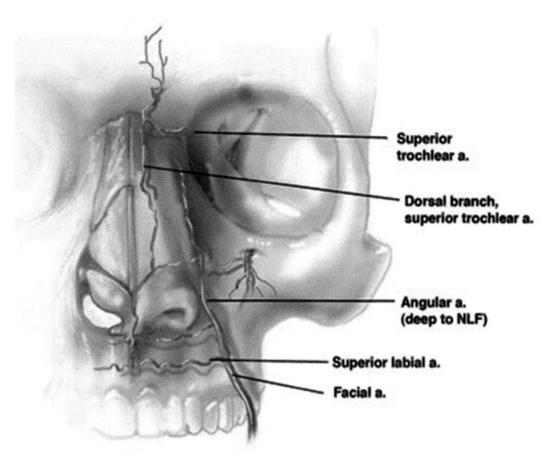

Fig. 3. Arterial anatomy of the face. Although not drawn to scale, this illustration highlights internal carotid artery branches and external carotid artery branches, showing the extensive anastomoses between vascular territories in the face's nasal region. Filler product has been carried in these anastomotic vessels from the perioral area to the periorbital area, and vice versa. Note that the facial artery has several known branch distribution types. NLF, nasolabial fold. (*From* DeLorenzi C. Complications of injectable fillers, part 2: vascular complications. Aesthetic Surg J. 2014;34(4):594; with permission.)

successful results; therefore, it is a promising method to correct these defects.[58–60]

Fat is an ideal filler because of the natural integration into tissues, being autologous, and perfect biocompatibility. Fat is also an active and a dynamic tissue that is composed of various cell types, including adipocytes, fibroblasts, myocytes, preadipocytes, and endothelial cells.[61–63]

Adipose-derived stem cells (ASCs), the same as other mesenchymal stem cells, have the potential for differentiation. In comparison with bone marrow-derived stem cells, ASCs have a greater yield upon isolation and a higher rate of proliferation in culture when.[64–66] Because of these features and owing to the simplicity of harvesting of these cells in large amounts with minor donor site morbidity, ASCs have been considered to be promising for application in regenerative therapies.[64,67]

Fat Harvesting

In 1987, Coleman introduced a novel technique for fat harvesting. His technique minimized the rate of complications from transferring of fat during liposuction was composed of 3 steps: manual lipoaspiration under low pressure, centrifugation for 3 minutes at 3400 rpm, and reinjection in 3 dimensions. Despite some technical modifications, Coleman technique remained as the gold standard for lipoplasty and lipofilling.[68] Nevertheless, owing to the variability of lipofilling results, it is necessary to optimize the procedure. The long-term results of fat grafting are often unsatisfactory because the partial absorption (up to 70% of the volume of the fat graft) is unpredictable. Previously, resorption rates of 30% to 70% per year have been reported.[69] Therefore, with regard to the unpredictability of success rates of autologous

Table 1
Summary of literature review

Authors (Year)	Title	Application of Fat Grafting	Study Duration	Total No. of Patients and No. Who Underwent 1, 2, or 3 Sessions; (Mean No. of Sessions)	No. of Men/No. Of Women	Mean Age, Years (Range)	Mean Injection Volume, mL (Range)	Mean Follow-up, Months (Range)	Primary Results	Key Contributions	Comments by Authors of the Present Study
Kao et al,[18] 2016	Microautologous Fat Transplantation for Primary Augmentation Rhinoplasty: Long-term Monitoring of 198 Asian Patients	Primary augmentation rhinoplasty for aesthetic purposes	4 y	198 patients; 126 (1 session) 70 (2 sessions) 2 (3 sessions); (1.4)	18/180	45.5 (26–58)	3.4 (2.0–5.5)	19 (6–42)	Overall satisfaction rate of 63.1%	First article to describe a large series of patients who underwent fat grafting in aesthetic primary augmentation rhinoplasty with MAFT	MAFT is appropriate for primary augmentation rhinoplasty for aesthetic purposes
Duskova et al (2004)	Augmentation by Autologous Adipose Tissue in Cleft Lip and Nose. Final Esthetic Touches in Clefts: Part I	Reconstruction in cleft lip and nose to supplement a hypertrophic scarred lip and nasal columella	NS	5 patients; 3 (1 session) 1 (2 sessions) (3 sessions) (2)	1/4	NS (26–38)	4.3 (3–6)	22 (NS)	All 5 patients have pleasing results	Described augmentation of the upper lip and columella by fat grafting is minimally invasive and results in physiologic shapes for the upper lip, nasal columella, and nasolabial angle	Small study but with promising results

Cárdenas et al,[14] 2007	Refinement of Rhinoplasty with Lipoinjection	As an adjunct to open rhinoplasty	2 y, 3 mo	78 patients 78 (1 session) (1)	7/71	NS (14–56)	NS (1–3)	15 (1–36)	Results of 68 patients considered excellent, 9 good, 1 unsatisfactory	Determined that fat grafting can be applied to refine open rhinoplasty	Concludes that fat grafting is an adjunct procedure with open rhinoplasty
Monreal,[1] 2011	Fat Grafting to the Nose: Personal Experience With 36 Patients	Primary augmentation, treatment of deformities after rhinoplasty, and in conjunction with rhinoplasty	3 y, 3 mo	36 patients 33 (1 session) 2 (2 sessions) (1.1)	NS	NS	Harvested 3–12 mL for lipoimplantation; 6–12 mL when combined with rhinoplasty	7 (NS-14)	80% (good to high) patient satisfaction, especially for deformities after rhinoplasty	Identified nasal danger zones and emphasized the importance of using an 18G, blunt injection needle	Only 18 of 36 patients (50%) presented for aesthetic purposes
Clauser et al (2011)	Structural Fat Grafting: Facial Volumetric Restoration in Complex Reconstructive Surgery	Volumetric restoration in complex reconstructive surgery	4 y, 5 mo	23 patients NA (NA)	NS	NS	3.4 NS	NS	Good results and improvements in facial morphology, function, shape, and volume	Demonstrated the importance of structural fat grafting in facial volumetric restoration in complex reconstructive surgery	Only 23 of 57 fat grafting procedures were discussed
Baptista et al,[3] 2013	Correction of Sequelae of Rhinoplasty by Lipofilling	To treat rhinoplasty sequelae, saddle nose, and sequelae of lateral osteotomy sequelae	4 y	20 patients 18 (1 session) 2 (2 sessions) (1.1)	NS	53 (NS)	2.1 (1–6)	NS (18–24)	18 patients satisfied to very satisfied, 2 required second rhinoplasty	Determined that lipofilling could be a simple and reliable alternative to correct imperfections following rhinoplasty	Correction of sequelae of rhinoplasty in 20 patients

(continued on next page)

Table 1
(continued)

Authors (Year)	Title	Application of Fat Grafting	Study Duration	Total No. of Patients and No. Who Underwent 1, 2, or 3 Sessions; (Mean No. of Sessions)	No. of Men/No. Of Women	Mean Age, Years (Range)	Mean Injection Volume, mL (Range)	Mean Follow-up, Months (Range)	Primary Results	Key Contributions	Comments by Authors of the Present Study
Erol[30] 2014	Microfat Grafting in Nasal Surgery	As microfat transplantation in patients with secondary nasal deformities (group 1 slight irregularities; group 2, marked irregularities; group 3, severe deformities)	5 y	313 patients: 264 group 1 patients (1–3 sessions); 38 group 2 patients (3–6 sessions); 11 group 3 patients (6–16 sessions) (NA)	27/286	25.7 NS	0.3–0.8 mL for minimal irregularities; 1–6 mL for major irregularities	NS (12–60)	Autologous microfat injection is safe and effective for correcting slight irregularities of the nose	Demonstrated that microfat grafting is effective for correcting minor irregularities of the nasal skin and is appropriate for patients who cannot undergo revision rhinoplasty	Multiple injections may be necessary for correction of nasal irregularities
Nguyen et al (2014)	Autologous Fat Grafting and Rhinoplasty	For correction of rhinoplasty sequelae	6 y	20 patients (1 session) 2 (2 sessions) (1.1)	NS	53 NS	2.1 (1–6)	NS (18–24)	18/20 patients satisfied to very satisfied	Emphasized the importance of using a 21G, 0.8-mm injection cannula vs an 18G, 1.2 mm cannula	Relatively small study size to address correcting the sequelae of rhinoplasty
Huang (2015)	Does Sensation Return to the Nasal Tip After Microfat Grafting?	Evaluation of severity of numbness in the nasal tip after fat grafting	4 y	30 patients 30 (1 session) (1)	0/30	20 (20–45)					

Abbreviations: NA, not applicable; NS, not stated.

From Kao W-P, Lin Y-N, Lin T-Y, et al. Microautologous fat transplantation for primary augmentation rhinoplasty: long-term monitoring of 198 Asian patients. Aesthet Surg J. 2016;36(6):651–2; with permission.

fat grafting, physicians are unable to select the perfect method for harvesting and transferring fat grafts.[55,69,70] The Coleman technique seems to be standard and favorable for these purposes, though it suffers from some limitations. First, owing to damage caused during the aspiration and centrifugation steps, the number of fat cells decreases; second, cells in direct contact with well-vascularized tissues need to be infiltrated.[71] Third, it is an operator-dependent and time-consuming technique for less experienced surgeons. Many attempts were made toward the alteration of the Coleman technique to improve the survival of the injected fat, atraumatic fat harvesting, fat washing for the removal of inflammatory mediators, incubating fat grafts with different bioactive substances, and centrifugation of fat grafts can be used.[40]

The main techniques for fat harvesting are suction aspiration, syringe aspiration, and surgical excision.[40] Recent experimental and clinical surveys have advocated the direct fat excision overaspiration. In their study, a fat cylinder graft was introduced by Fagrell and colleagues. In this technique, fat is drilled out in cores by a punching device.[72,73] In another study, a core graft for block grafting was suggested by Qin and colleagues,[72,74] because in this technique, the structure and viability of the harvested fat tissues are preserved without impairment of the adipocytes. Pu and colleagues[72,75] observed damaged adipocyte function in conventional liposuction aspirates relative to fresh fatty tissue samples and syringe aspiration of fat. Compared with syringe aspiration, lipoaspiration at a low negative pressure may yield fat faster, particularly when a large volume of fat is required. The high vacuum pressures of conventional liposuction may give rise to functional disruption in the majority of adipocytes.[72,76] Cannula size is one of the other main factors affecting the viability of harvested fat.[77] Using large-bore cannulas in the excisional method and fat harvesting can decrease the incidence of cellular rupture and maintain the native tissue structure. Campbell and colleagues,[78] however, found that there is a reverse correlation between damage to cells and the diameter of the instrument used to extract fat. Additionally, Erdim and colleagues[79] reported that using a 6-mm cannula instead of a thinner (4 or 2 mm) cannula can enhance adipocyte viability. Described in the technique proposed by Coleman[80] for fat harvesting, fat is manually suctioned with a 3-mm, 2-hole cannula linked to a 10-mL syringe by removing the plunger. The cannula is then pushed through the harvesting site during digital manipulation by the surgeon to draw back on the syringe plunger and create a gentle negative pressure.[80]

Fat is naturally deposited in different parts of the body. The most suitable site for fat harvesting is identified by the surgeon after a precise examination of the patient. One of the most common sites for fat harvesting is the abdomen, followed by the trochanteric region (saddlebags) and the inside of the thighs and knees.[81,82]

The are 2 methods for harvesting of fat grafts: a wet and a dry method. In the wet method, which was described by Klein and colleagues[72,83] in 1993, the donor site is injected with a fluid (Klein's) solution composed of 0.9% NaCl, epinephrine, and a local anesthetic. Hydrodissection and enlargement of the target fat layer are reported indications of the wet method. Low shear stress has been demonstrated to improve graft survival and, in fact, is a factor affecting adipocyte viability.[84] An alternative to a wet method is the dry method, which is done without the tumescent fluid. However, this method may result in a greater need for analgesics.[83]

Fat Processing

Sedimentation, filtering, washing, and centrifugation are methods commonly used for the preparation of fat grafts. Lipoaspirate is composed of adipocytes, collagen fibers, blood, and debris; therefore, fat processing is a necessary step in fat grafting. These components often result in inflammation at the recipient site and cause damage to the fat graft.[40] The effects of fat processing with the fat graft preparation methods mentioned create no significant differences in fat retention. However, unlike centrifugation, filtration led to nodule formation.[85,86] After centrifugation, 3 layers are observed; the upper layer consists of lipids and can be poured off using absorbent material. The middle layer includes fatty tissue, and the lower layer is composed of blood, tissue fluid, and local anesthetic, which is ejected from the base of syringe. For adipose tissue grafting, the middle layer is routinely used.[87–89]

Fat Injection

Cannulas with small gauges are believed to minimize trauma to the recipient site and decrease the risks of bleeding, hematoma formation, and poor graft oxygen diffusion.[72] Because revascularization starts at the periphery, the ischemic time is longer in the center of the graft.[90] Accordingly, fat injection is preferred to be performed in multiple small-volume sessions rather than only 1 session.

There is a direct relationship between the nature of the recipient site and the selection of cannula size. Infiltration with cannulas of at least 2.5 mm in diameter can increase the viability of adipose tissue,[77] whereas various needle gauges did not confer significant differences in cell viability.[79] To successfully gain the prolonged survival of autologous fat, it is necessary to use small injections of grafts (thinner than 2–3 mm). An adipose tissue graft obtains its nutrition through plasmatic imbibition from approximately 1.5 mm of its vascularized edge. Hence, fat grafts with a diameter of less than 3 mm can have a better long-term survival rate. In a number of patients, they have remained in place and stable for 10 to 20 years.[57,91–93]

In a rabbit face model, the placement of fat grafts was investigated in varied tissue planes. The results of morphometric and histologic measurements of transplanted fat grafts suggested the higher survival of fat grafts, especially when placing in supramuscular layer rather than subcutaneous or submuscular layer. These findings verify that fat graft placement in varied tissue planes is favorable for better clinical achievements.[53,94] Less fibrous fat has better flow characteristics, allowing for smoother infiltration. Thus, recognition of the flow characteristics of the fat being injected helps to avoid deformities and ensure that samples of similar quality are used symmetrically.[21]

Role of Adipose-Derived Stem Cells

ASCs, similar to bone marrow–derived stem cells, are able to differentiate into several mesodermal tissue types and also indicate similar expression of surface protein marker.[67,95] Meanwhile, unlike bone marrow-derived stem cells, ASCs can readily be attained using a standard wet liposuction technique under local anesthesia, without the need for expansion in culture.[67,96] For these reasons, ASCs have received attention for their application in cell-based therapies involving the repair and regeneration of damaged tissue. Stem cells isolated from lipoaspirates have the ability to differentiate in vitro into adipocytes, osteocytes, chondrocytes, myocytes, caryomioblasts, and neurons.[97–99] For isolation of ASC, there are 2 methods: the first method is based on a mechanical and enzymatic procedure,[100] and the second method is exclusively mechanical.[101]

Cell-assisted lipotransfer is a new approach to autologous tissue transfer, first introduced by Matsumoto and colleagues in 2006.[102] Indeed, cell-assisted lipotransfer is the simultaneous transplantation of ASCs and aspirated fat. In this method, ASCs are applied to maximize the effectiveness of autologous lipoinjection, that is, to attain a higher survival rate and the persistence of transplanted fat, as well as to minimize complications from lipoinjection, including fibrosis, pseudocyst formation, and calcification.[102]

Adipose tissue has lately been recognized as a source of ASCs or processed lipoaspirate cells, which are abundant in the lower abdomen and inner thigh. These 2 parts of the body are thought to be the better donor sites for adult ASCs relative to other typical donor sites. This finding means that fat graft not only can serve as a filler, but also can improve the quality of aged and scarred skin.[53,103,104] Adipose tissue has been considered as a source of stem cells, which are able to differentiate into many other mature cells.[105–107]

In fat grafting, the regenerative attributes of mesenchymal stem cells has been applied for the treatment of many complications, including long-term ulcerations, skin atrophy owing to radiotherapy, and burn healing.[89,108–112] Using fat in syndromes such as Raynaud phenomenon and unilateral vocal cord paralysis has also been reported.[113–116]

METHODS

Cárdenas and Carvajal[14] presented a procedure using lipoinjection for the refinement of rhinoplasty in 2006. From 78 patients who participated in this study, 61 and 17 were selected for primary and secondary rhinoplasties, respectively, with a follow-up time of 1 to 36 month(s). Before the initiation of open rhinoplasty and at the beginning of the procedure, 1 to 3 mL of autologous fat was injected to the nose through small incisions (0.5 cm). After the amount of fat was determined based on individual patient needs, it was placed in the radix, dorsum sides, and supratip regions. At the end of the rhinoplasty, the fat was injected subcutaneously over the osseocartilaginous framework using a 1-mL syringe. The fat was used as a thin layer of soft tissue to thicken the covering skin and aid in concealing minor imperfections. No minor deformities were observed, and in all the patients, the quality of the skin was improved. The authors reached the conclusion that refinement of rhinoplasty by injecting fat into the nose can serve as a rapid, simple, and inexpensive procedure for obtaining long-term symmetric contours on the nasal dorsum.[14]

In 2011, Juan Monreal[1] performed an investigation on 33 patients with nasal deformity. In his study, 15 cases were injected with 6- to 12-mL fat grafts, instead of cartilage or prosthesis, on the nose to complete deficient bone. However, in 18 cases, 3- to 12-mL fat grafts were used for patients with or without previous surgery as the unique method of improving nasal aesthetics. For the 33 cases, 36 procedures were undertaken, with a maximum follow-up period of 14 months (mean, 7 months). Changes in volume and shape of the nose, aesthetic improvement, and patient satisfaction were analyzed by comparing preoperative with postoperative control photographs. The results of nasal lipoimplantations showed that patients with a previous surgery had a bit more swelling and ecchymosis than those who refused the primary surgical rhinoplasty. After 4 to 5 months, none of the patients observed alterations in contour or volume. Because of the use of the small volumes of fat, it was difficult to determine the percentage of final graft take, which was 60% and 75% in cases who refused primary and secondary surgical rhinoplasty, respectively. Patient satisfaction was estimated to be good to excellent in 80% of cases, especially in cases of postrhinoplasty deformity. Monreal concluded that fillers or fat grafts cannot be a substitute for a surgical technique, and their results will never be more favorable. However, autologous fat grafting can serve as a first-line nonsurgical alternative to the reconstruction of nasal shape, particularly for patients who refuse primary and secondary surgical rhinoplasties and accept the limitations inherent to the technique. The aesthetic nasal and paranasal units can be considered as a whole or as aesthetic subunits separately, if necessary. Moreover, surgical rhinoplasty can be combined with lipoimplantation in different areas of nose, including the dorsum, radix, glabella, or premaxillary, to change the volume and shape of these areas without using cartilage grafts or solid prostheses.[1]

In 2012, Baptista and colleagues[3] assessed "correction of sequelae of rhinoplasty by lipofilling." A total of 20 patients participated in their study and received an injection of 1 to 6 mL of adipose tissue to the nose. Based on their results, surgical sequela was corrected in 15 cases after primary rhinoplasty and in 5 cases after secondary rhinoplasty, with an interval of at least 1 year after the first or last procedure. They applied different cannula sizes for fat collection and injection, that is, 11G (3 mm) and 7G (1.7 mm) cannula in 10 patients and 14G (2 mm) and 21G (0.8 mm) in another 10 patients, for harvesting and injecting, respectively. Based on the location of the nasal defect, the insertion points were in the glabellar region at the base of the ala nasi or the columella. The injection plane is normally performed in contact with the periosteum, but the recent use of microcannula allows for injections in the superficial musculoaponeurotic system or in the direct subdermal

plane. Patient follow-up appointments were at 2 weeks, 2 months, and 18 months. The results were evaluated based on patients' satisfaction and surgeons' comments with regard to comparison of preoperative and postoperative photos at 18 months. "In patients who have undergone multiple operations, microinjection of adipose tissue can be a simple and reliable alternative for correction of imperfections following rhinoplasty."[3]

In 2014, Erol[30] conducted a research of autologous microfat grafting in nasal surgery. In his 5-year survey, microfat grafting was applied to treat 313 patients with secondary nasal malformation and minor skin deformities or severe nasal skin damage. Extra harvested fat at each patient's first injection session was cryopreserved for later injection. The minimal malformations were corrected by the injection of 0.3 to 0.8 mL of microfat during each session. However, for the maximal deformities or defects, 1 to 6 mL of microfat was used for each session. The most frequent areas for fat harvesting were the abdomen and flanks, followed by the trochanteric region, buttocks, or medial thigh. Fat was obtained through a small incision from patients under general anesthesia via a 10-mL syringe and 3-mm cannula; local anesthetic was not used for donor sites. Sealed Luer-Lok syringes were then centrifuged at 3000 rpm for 3 minutes. The upper (containing liquid lipid) and lower (containing aqueous) layers were discarded, and 1 g of first-generation cephalosporin was added to each 100 g of centrifuged fat tissue.

Protocol for Freezing and Thawing

After the injection of the required amount of fat or tissue cocktail, the excessive fat was cryopreserved. Samples were transferred to sterile tubes of different sizes (10, 20, or 50 mL), labeled, and frozen at −196°C in a liquid nitrogen tank. The cryopreserved graft samples were first placed in a UF 601 medical refrigerator (−80°C; Electrolux, Stockholm, Sweden), and then were taken from the medical refrigerator and transferred to a standard refrigerator (−15°C) 12 hours before subsequent procedures and finally thawed gradually at room temperature for 1 hour before injection. There are many controversies over fat freezing, and some researchers refuse to use frozen fat.[8]

The patient's nasal area was marked for injection while the patient was standing. The recipient sites received a local anesthesia, consisting of a mixture of 0.5% bupivacaine (20 mL), adrenaline (0.50 mg), physiologic serum (30 mL), and triamcinolone acetonide (20 mg), to diminish posttreatment edema and ecchymosis and also to create vessel vasoconstriction to minimize the risk of microembolism.

Injections were carried out depending on the thickness of the skin with an intravenous cannula (22G or 24G). The correction of minor malformations was performed with the injection (1–3 times) of 0.3 to 0.8 mL of cryopreserved microfat graft material. However, major malformations or defects were corrected by the injection (3–6 times) of 1 to 6 mL of the graft material. Meanwhile, for patients with severe nasal irregularities with damaged skin, cryopreserved microfat graft material was injected at 2-month intervals (6–16 times).

Repeated injections of the cryopreserved fat were conducted, if required. Intradermal or subcutaneous injection of tiny amounts of fat was performed depending on the injection site. Patients who required repeated injections received a local anesthetic and evaluated by comparing their pretreatment and posttreatment photographs. For patients with minor irregularities, 1 to 3 injections of microfat were necessary, whereas cases with multiple and severe irregularities required 3 to 6 injections. The patients were highly satisfied with the injections. Another group of patients who had severe traumatic skin damage needed 6 to 16 injections for reconstruction. Each patient's skin damage was repaired after repeated injections. Autologous microfat grafting seems to be a safe and efficient procedure for the correction of not only minor irregularities of nasal skin, but also severely damaged skin on the nose.[30]

Kornstein and Nikfarjam[21] published an article entitled, "Fat Grafting to the Forehead/Glabella/Radix Complex and Pyriform Aperture: Aesthetic and Anti-Aging Implications" in 2015. Participants in their study were divided into 2 groups: the first group included patients who underwent fat grafting alone (FG group; n = 26), and the second group consisted of patients who underwent fat grafting plus rhinoplasty (FG + R group; n = 19). The mean follow-up of the first and second groups was 3.3 and 5.2 years, respectively. Tumescent fluid was used to infiltrate donor sites. Also, the harvested fat samples were centrifuged. The main objective was to achieve a homogeneous paste with the ability to be readily and predictably injected. To provide cannula access, a 16G needle was used instead of incisions. Subsequently, fat was injected in small aliquots using a 17G side port, bullet-tip cannula. The cannula tip was placed to a depth of palpating bone. Next, tiny aliquots of fat were injected to preserve close contact with sufficient vascular supply, the same as skin grafting. Fat (virtually 20 cm^3) was then injected into the lower forehead and nasofrontal regions until the achievement of aesthetic end point of a lateral-to-lateral and cranial-to-caudal gentle convexity. The mean nasofrontal angle in the 2 groups (FG and FG + R) decreased by 2.0° ($P = .005$ and $P = .011$, respectively). However, the nasolabial angle increased by 2.3° ($P = .006$) in the FG group and by 6.0° ($P = .026$) in the FG + R group. Fat grafting to the forehead–glabella–radix complex and pyriform aperture can act as a reliable technique for favorable modification of both the nasofrontal and nasolabial angles. This method helps to improve the interaction between the nose and the adjacent facial features, which ultimately maximizes the overall aesthetics.

Numerous techniques are available for fat injection and are discussed in various investigations. In a previous study of 198 Asian patients undergoing augmentation rhinoplasty, Kao and colleagues in 2016 used MAFT-GUN, an adjustable device applied for delivering different sizes of fat parcels.[18] He augmented these particles to the nose from nasal tip to an area approximately 15 mm above the interconthal line. The total volume of fat was injected into upper, middle, and lower zones on the nasal dorsum.

Initially, fat was harvested from the lower abdomen by injecting tumescent fluid into the harvesting area. The volumes of lipoaspirate and tumescent fluid was approximately equal, to ensure that fat represented a major proportion of the lipoaspirate. To mitigate damage to the lipoaspirate, a 10-mL syringe plunger, which was connected to a liposuction cannula, was pulled back to approximately 2 to 3 mL for preserving a negative pressure of 270 to 330 mm Hg. Lipoaspirates were purified by centrifugation at approximately $1200 \times g$ for 3 minutes. In this method, owing to environmental exposure and manual manipulation, graft contamination was minimized. Separation of the lipoaspirate into layers was facilitated by centrifugation. The upper and middle layers contained oil from ruptured fat cells and purified fat, respectively, whereas the lower layer was composed of blood, cellular debris, and fluid. A transducer was then used to transfer the purified fat into a 1-mL Luer-slip syringe. The purified fat-containing syringe was loaded into a MAFT-Gun, which was connected to an 18G blunt-tip cannula. Fat parcels of 0.0067 mL (1/150 mL) to 0.0056 mL (1/180 mL), with each trigger deployment, were transferred by the device set by adjusting a dial. At the nasal tip, a single puncture incision was induced with a #11 scalpel blade, and it was infiltrated with 2% lidocaine HCl (0.3–0.5 mL) with a 1:50,000 concentration of epinephrine. Subsequently, fat was transferred by depressing the trigger, while pulling out the

MAFT-Gun. Fat was carefully injected into 2 to 3 layers of the nasal dorsum, that is, from the deep areolar plane to the vascular/fibromuscular plane to the subcutaneous areolar plane. During MAFT, the surgeon used their nondominant hand to apply downward traction to 3 zones of the nose, first on the middle third of the nose while grafting the upper third and second on the lower third of the nose (the nasal tip) while grafting the middle third. Finally, after transferring fat to the nasal tip, the insertion point was closed using a nonabsorbable suture (6-0). The rate of fat retention was estimated to be 50% or less at 6 months postoperatively. After monitoring for an average of 19 months, patients were satisfied with the outcome. The satisfaction rate for those who underwent 1 session of MAFT was acceptable, but it was excellent for those who underwent 2 or 3 sessions.[18]

In a pilot study by Lin and collogues in 2017,[113] nasal dorsum contouring using fat injection was analyzed. In this study, 13 patients were evaluated and received fat injection using a MAFT-Gun for the first time. The patients were 12 females and 1 male, and their mean age was 34.03 ± 7.28 years (range, 22–47 years). Reconstructions of 3-dimensional photography images, which were taken before fat injection and 3 months later, were performed with 3dMDvultus software. In total, 26 scans were obtained from all the patients and were analyzed. The results were reported as mean $\pm$ standard deviation. The amount of fat injected for nasal dorsum augmentation was 1.67 ± 0.95 mL (range, 0.6–3.3 mL). Based on calculation using the 3dMDvultus software, the volume changes were 0.74 ± 0.42 mL and 0.74 ± 0.43 mL for the first and second measurements, respectively. Also, the intraobserver consistency measured by Cronbach $\alpha = 0.96$ ($P<.001$) was high. Based on the 3-dimensional images, the mean volume change and the mean retention rate was 0.74 ± 0.42 mL (range, 0.21–1.53 mL) and 44.54%, respectively.

The impact of fat grafting on edema and ecchymoses in primary rhinoplasty was studied by Gabrick and coworkers[117] in 2019. They applied Telfa-rolling technique for fat processing. Using a 19G needle and 1-mL syringes, the fat was injected into the deep surface of the periosteum of the nasolabial fold and medial canthal areas. The harvested fat averaged 3.7 mL and ranged from 1 to 21 mL. All patients had autologous fat grafting to these areas (100%) and some to additional facial regions. The researchers came to the conclusion that autologous fat grafting is a helpful supplementary method for primary rhinoplasty.

Furthermore, in this method, resolution of postoperative bruising occurs rapidly in the immediate postoperative period.[117]

FILLERS

According to American Society of Plastic surgeons' reports, filler procedures increased from 650,000 in 2000 to 2.3 million procedures in 2014.[20] The role of fillers in nasal reshaping continues to be explored and filler injection is not considered standard of care for the long-term management of nasal defects. Therefore, there are great controversies surrounding this subject.[20]

In a 20-year retrospective study in 1986, Webster and associates[118] introduced a procedure, microdroplet silicone injection into the nasal bridge, for the correction of postsurgical nasal defects. Although favorable results were recorded in the study, many physicians have remained skeptical about silicone injections owing to atrocious complications reported from the 1960s and 1970s.[43]

In 1981, bovine collagen injections became popular among cosmetic surgeons, starting with Zyderm collagen (Allergan, Inc, Irvine, CA). From that time on, various new products entered the market. One of the most popularized products is hyaluronic acid (HA), so-called hyaluronan, which is a high-molecular-weight linear polysaccharide containing alternating D-glucuronic acid and N-acetylglucosamine.

During an analysis of bovine vitreous in 1934, Meyer and Palmer[119] described HA as a natural sugar found in the skin and tissues. They also explained that this naturally occurring substance performs not only physical (such as lubrication) functions, but also and chemical functions, which act as essential vital substrates for numerous biological processes, such as fertility, embryogenesis, morphogenesis, cellular migration, inflammation, and wound healing.[120] HA in its natural state is a perfect filler material, but has an extremely short half-life.[121–128] To retard natural turnover and enhance its lifespan, manufacturers have attempted to modify the chemistry of HA by crosslinking chains using different dispersants such as 1,4-butanediol diglyceryl ether.[129] Minimal modification of the material enabled manufacturers to produce HA products that can be well-tolerated by the immune system, as well as are durable and nonreactive.

The initial attempts at manufacturing HA were based on the use of animal-sourced raw materials and plagued by protein contamination issues.[130] Accordingly, Lancefield groups A and C *Streptococcus equi* subspecies *zooepidemicus*, which naturally produce a pure hyaluronate mucoid capsule, were used for the development of commercial sources of hyaluronates. Hence, bacterial broths were a suitable source for the production of large quantities of relatively pure hyaluronates because they needed only purification of quite simple bacterial protein contaminants instead of the complex proteins that contaminated mammalian or avian sources. Serious attempts were made to extend HA lifespan in tissues by development of products with more crosslinks between chains, but it decreased tissue tolerance owing to increased immune-mediated adverse events. Therefore, a balance is required whereby natural HA chemical structure was increased enough from its natural state, to minimize its susceptibility to breakdown. Even though HA is recognized as the dominant filler product for volumizing tissues, there are many dermal filler materials.[10] Silicone oils, poly(methyl methacrylate) microspheres, polyacrylamide, and other materials, alone or in combination with resorbable components, are examples of permanent dermal fillers.[131–136]

There are different physical features associated with injectables. Viscosity and elasticity are 2 important attributes in a filler. Viscosity is a measure of the gel's ability to resist sheering forces.[16,137] In other words, it is resistance ability of a material to a pressure applied to it, which denotes that it is less probable to spread. Products with low viscosity are more readily spread, whereas products with high viscosity have tendency to stay put, which allows for more precise sculpting. Elasticity refers to the material's ability to resist malformation when force is applied. Fillers with high elasticity offer more lift and support, and require smaller amounts to achieve correction. Fillers having both features, viscosity and elasticity, are more appropriate for nonsurgical rhinoplasty. The 2 features have also investigated in 6 cross-linked HA products, including Restylane, Restylane Sub-Q (Q-Med, Uppsala, Sweden), Perlane, Juvederm Ultra, Juvederm Ultra Plus, and Juvederm Voluma (Allergan, Pringy, France) and also calcium hydroxylapatite (CaHA) and CaHA lidocaine mixture, according to the guidelines provided by the US Food and Drug Administration.[16] Based on the data from this investigation, the products were divided into 3 groups of high, medium, and low viscosity and elasticity. The first (high) group included undiluted Radiesse. Radiesse mixed with 0.3% lidocaine and 3 HA products such as Restylane, Perlane, and Restylane Sub-Q (unavailable in the United States) were in the second (medium) group. Juvederm Ultra, Juvederm Ultra Plus, and Juvederm Voluma (unavailable in the United States) were other HA

products included in the third (low) group. The viscosity and elasticity of each product can be modified by its dilution with lidocaine or saline, which is a very popularized strategy. Overdilution may, however, result in the need for more injection of product at the target site. Contour alteration with a very small amount of filler is advantageous. Therefore, care should be taken about diluting the natural product of the dermal filler because the injection of larger amounts of materials may cause a higher occurrence of vascular complications.[2]

In a filler, hydrophilicity is an important factor that is needs to be considered. Although being shown to be desirable in filler rhinoplasty, the hydrophilic effect of HA products may clinically be disadvantageous. For instance, the expansion arises from the leakage of water into the tissues may enhance the potential for compression of dermal and subdermal vessels, which is likely results in vascular compromise. Among the HA products, Restylane and Perlane have less hydrophilicity than Juvederm Ultra and Ultra Plus.[138]

For nonsurgical rhinoplasty, CaHA can serve as a filler of choice. Its longevity (averaging roughly 9–12 months) and moldability are very similar to those of a perfect filler, particularly for this application. However, the replacement of HA products with hyaluronidase makes them appealing to aesthetic physicians who had less experience in nonsurgical rhinoplasty.[2]

Successful injection of CaHA (Radiesse, Merz, San Mateo, CA) for the correction of the internal nasal valve collapse has previously been reported.[139] Radiesse is a suspension of CaHA microspheres (30%; 25–45 μm) in glycerin, carboxymethyl cellulose, and water mixture. Owing to similarity with the mineral portion of human bone and teeth, CaHA is fully biocompatible.[140] Radiesse was first approved as a radiologic marker and for use in vocal fold augmentation, and later in 2006, it was approved by FDA for cosmetic applications (**Tables 2** and **3**).[43]

Dermal fillers are generally classified into reversible and irreversible classes,[141] rather than temporary versus permanent. HA fillers are reversible dermal fillers because HA-based reversible dermal fillers may be fully eliminated with the use of hyaluronidase.[141–149] Using HA in the treatment of saddle nose can offer patients an improved cosmetic appearance in place of, or preceding, definitive surgical nasal reconstruction (**Table 4**).[20]

Complications

As with other techniques, fat grafting and injecting fillers are associated with some complications,

Table 2
Dermal fillers approved by the FDA since 1981

	Irreversible	Synthetic		Reversible — Natural Source	
Major Component	Polymethyl methacrylate (PMMA)[a]	Hydroxylapatite[b]	Poly-L-lactic acid (PLLA)[c]	Hyaluronic acid[d]	Collagen[e]
Year first approved	2006	2006	2004	2003	1981
Brand name (manufacturer)	Artefill (Suneva Medical, San Diego, CA)	Radiesse (Merz Aesthetics, San Mateo, CA)	Sculptra (Valeant, Bridgewater, NJ)	Restylane, Perlane (Q-Med [Uppsala, Sweden]/Valeant [Bridgewater, NJ]); Hylaform, Hylaform Plus (Genzyme Biosurgery, Ridgefield, NJ); Juvéderm30, Juvéderm30HV, Juvéderm24HV (Allergan, Irvine, CA); Elevess (Anika Therapeutics, Bedford, MA)	Zyderm, Zyplast (Allergan); Cosmoderm, Cosmoplast (Allergan); Evolence (ColBar Life Science, Mattawan, MI)

This table is not a complete listing of all products available.

Abbreviation: FDA, US Food and Drug Administration.

[a] Poly(methyl methacrylate) (PMMA): a synthetic nonbiodegradable polymer also used in bone cement and synthetic intraocular lenses. It is formulated in 40-micron microspheres suspended in bovine collagen.

[b] Calcium hydroxylapatite: mineral typically found in teeth and bone. Reconstituted as a gel suspension and injected. Lasts approximately 18 mo.

[c] Poly-L-lactic acid: a slowly biodegradable polymer that has been used in suture materials for many years. Results may last up to 2 y, depending on site of injection.

[d] Hyaluronic acid: polysaccharide that binds water and is sourced from avian (eg, rooster combs) or streptococcal bacteria. The polysaccharide is cross-linked to resist degradation, extending its durability from 6 to 18 mo, depending on formulation and region injected.

[e] Collagen: protein derived from cow (bovine) or human cells, lasting 3 to 4 mo, the shortest duration of any of the dermal fillers. Collagen products have been discontinued and are no longer available.

From DeLorenzi C. Complications of injectable fillers, part I. Aesthet Surg J. 2013;33(4):562; with permission.

Table 3
Paradigm of injectables and their physical attributes G′ and N′

G′: elasticity coefficient. Ability to resist deformation from pressure; higher indicates more lift with less volume		N′: viscosity coefficient. Ability to resist sheering forces; less diffusion into tissue
High G′ and high N′	Medium G′ and N′	Low G′ and N′
CaHA: Radiesse	CaHA with lidocaine and HA: Restylane, Perlane, Restylane SubQ, Restylane Lyft	HA: Juvederm Ultra, Juvederm Ultra Plus, Juvederm Voluma, Belotero Balance
Less diffusion; precise sculpting		More diffusion; improved blending
Less volume needed for lift		More volume needed for lift

From Thomas WW, Bucky L, Friedman O. Injectables in the nose: facts and controversies. Facial Plast Surg Clin North Am. 2016;24(3):381; with permission.

including skin blanching, ecchymoses, delayed capillary refill, and dusky, bluish skin owing to necrosis and skin sloughs.[39] These complications mostly occur owing to injection methods, injectates, the anatomy of the zones to be injected, and the body's immune system. Cellulitis, swelling, pain, paresthesia, ecchymoses, hematoma and scar formation, shape and contour irregularities of area, and neighboring tissue damage are the most frequently occurring complications of harvesting fat.[82,162–166]

As mentioned elsewhere in this article, there are some complications with the location of injection, particularly with fillers and fat autologous grafts. Cyst formation and calcification in fat as well as necrosis and hypertrophy of fat occur mainly owing to the large amount of fat injection or injection to the area with low vascularization.[82,167–171] One of the most common complications is variable maintenance of fat and necessity for fat reinjection.[169,172] Although unpredictable, the durability of fat as a filler has been reported to be 10% to 80%.[173,174] This broad range of durability comes from various techniques for harvesting, processing, and injecting the fat; the characteristic and situation of donor site; and the site of host tissue.[75,175–177] Infection of the location of injection owing to nonsterile methods, erythema, and bleeding are other complications associated with harvesting fat.[168,178,179] Thus, sterile methods for harvesting, processing, and delivering the fat play an important role in avoiding complications. There are some reports on transmission of *Pseudomonas* infection via centrifuge sleeves.[53]

The most important complication in the face, especially nose, is the injection of materials to the vascular system (particularly in glabella) and to the nasolabial fold for supplying the nasal tip area. Indeed, fat can cause stasis in the vascular system and bring about a stroke or necrosis of the nasal tip. The movement of fat can also cause blindness and ocular thrombosis.[180,181] A devastating case of blindness owing to fat transplantation to the glabella has been reported.[182] Moreover, according to reports, patients have died from middle cerebral artery occlusion and ocular thrombosis and stroke owing to fat injection to the face.[183,184] Comparison of fat with fillers has revealed that vascular injuries from fat injection are more complicated because of the greater pressure and the larger volume used during injections.[185] It seems that vascular injuries arise from using sharp needles and high-pressure syringes[53]; therefore, aspiration before injection and the use of a blunt cannula, low-pressure syringes (1 mL), administration of vasoconstrictors (such as low-dose epinephrine), injecting a small volume of fat (using a MAFT-Gun), and avoiding sharp needles are important considerations.[186,187] Meanwhile, practitioners should be cautioned about the amount of hand pressure used during the injection to the glabella to avoid fat injection to the artery and subsequent retinal or cerebral artery obstruction.[47,49,181,188]

Sufficient knowledge of vascular anatomy of nose is very crucial and helps to preclude such phenomena. Migration of fat through the angular artery or dorsal nasal artery to the brain or in a retrograde direction, as a result of high-pressure injection, can cause blindness or brain stroke. In contrast, migration or stasis of fat in the dorsal nasal artery or angular artery or lateral nasal artery

Table 4
Clinical literature overview of use of dermal fillers in nonsurgical rhinoplasty

Reference	Filler/Procedure	Key Points of Study
Knapp and Vistnes,[150] 1985	Bovine collagen/surgical depressions resulting from rhinoplasty	Short-term filler may retain correction indefinitely
Webster et al,[118] 1986	Medical grade silicone/ injected subdermally for postrhinoplasty defects	347 patients/1937 treatments; recommended undercorrection because filler stimulates indigenous collagen growth.
Han et al,[151] 2006	Restylane (Q-Med, Uppsala, Sweden) coupled with autologous fibroblasts from harvested dermis/ augmentation rhinoplasty	11 patients; 10%–40% resorption in the first 6 mo in 6 patients; stabilization at 6 mo. Minor surgery rather than noninvasive as a result of epidermal flap necessary for harvesting. Used fibroblasts to increase longevity.
Beer,[152] 2006	Restylane/postrhinoplasty defect of nasal dorsum	Case report of 1 patient: safe, inexpensive, well-tolerated; mention of CaHA as alternative.
Becker,[153] 2008	Radiesse (Merz Aesthetics, San Mateo, CA)/Nonsurgical rhinoplasty	25 patients, 15 with previous surgical rhinoplasty; viable alternative to surgery; preferred CaHA caused by moldability and durability; mean patient satisfaction 7.9/10.0.
Rokhsar and Ciocon,[154] 2008	Radiesse/primary correction of nasal deformities	14 patients; no significant complications, high patient satisfaction.
de Lacerda and Zancanaro,[155] 2007	Porcine collagens and HAs/ filler rhinoplasty vs augmentation rhinoplasty	Filler rhinoplasty perhaps more accurate term than augmentation because of creating illusion of smaller nose through augmentation.
Cassuto,[156] 2009	Evolence (Ortho Dermatologics, Skillman, NJ)/nonsurgical rhinoplasty	12 patients; mean follow-up of 8 mo with stable correction.
Siclovan and Jomah,[157] 2009	Evolence/nasal deformities and postrhinoplasty irregularities	Correction for up to 1 y.
Humphrey et al,[138] 2009	HAs, CaHA, silicone review article	HA/CaHA safest available agents for nasal dorsum and sidewall deformities. Caution against filler in tip of nose.

(continued on next page)

Table 4 (continued)		
Reference	**Filler/Procedure**	**Key Points of Study**
Rivkin and Soliemanzadeh,[158] 2009	CaHA in nonsurgical rhinoplasty	4-y retrospective study of 385 patients (295 for follow-up); 46% required touch-up 2 mo after initial treatment; 28% touch-up 2–6 mo after initial treatment; 18% touch-up 6 mo to 1 y after initial treatment. Adverse events: prolonged erythema (more prevalent in postsurgical rhinoplasty patients) with 2 cases of partial skin necrosis and 6 cases of cellulitis.
Bray et al,[159] 2010	Restylane/nonsurgical nasal augmentation and postrhinoplasty asymmetry	Duration up to 18 mo; mention of CaHA to treat internal valve collapse.
Dayan and Kempiners,[160] 2005	Botulinum toxin either alone or with injectable fillers/nasal tip ptosis and acute nasolabial angle	5 units of botulinum toxin in depressor septi muscle bilaterally and 3 units into each levator labii superioris alaeque nasi muscle.
Monreal,[1] 2011	Autologous fat transfer/stand-alone correction or with surgical rhinoplasty	33 patients, 36 treatments; grafting to radix, glabella, pyriform aperture. Volume decrease first 15–30 d, stable thereafter. Duration unknown.
Kim and Ahn,[161] 2012	Radiesse/nonsurgical augmentation in Asian population	87 patients, 4 complications: 1 dorsal asymmetry (corrected), 1 overinjection of columella-labial angle causing intraoral submucosal nodule, 1 self-limited dermatitis, 1 inflammation/erythema at injection site; plane was subdermal with CaHA and intradermal with HA for tip.

From Jasin ME. Nonsurgical rhinoplasty using dermal fillers. Facial Plast Surg Clin North Am. 2013;21(2):242; with permission.

and its movement to the terminal arteries cause necrosis in the area supplied by these arteries.[1] In artery accidents, in which skin blanching lasts for a long period, repositioning the patient to the Trendelenburg position, using vasodilator pastes such as nitroglycerine, and rubbing the area with the hand is highly recommended.[53] Another important complication in the face the is formation of visible fat nodules owing to dorsal nasal thin skin; hence, the injection of small volumes of fat and fillers is necessary.[18] Nodules are typically produced when fat is injected too superficially.[189]

In case of blanching after 3 to 5 minutes, some surgeons suggest fat extrusion (**Table 5**).[18]

A knowledge of vascular anatomy of nose is crucial to prevent these phenomena. The migration of fat through the angular artery or dorsal nasal artery to the brain or in a retrograde direction, owing to high-pressure injection, could cause blindness or stroke. Although migration of fat or stasis of fat in the dorsal nasal artery, angular artery, or lateral nasal artery along with the moving to the terminal arteries could cause necrosis in the tissue supplied by these arteries.[1]

Table 5
Fat compared with HA injectable complications

	Fat	HA	*P* Value
Extent of occlusion: diffuse	86%, 19 of 22	39%, 5 of 13	.007
Best correct visual acuity (log conversion of Snellen chart) (SD)	2.6 (0.8) Higher is worse	1.4 (1.4)	.01
Long-term vision loss	100%, 9 of 9	43%, 3 of 7	.02
Cerebral lesions	46%, 10 of 22	8%, 1 of 13	.03
Site of injection	Glabella: 13 Nasolabial fold: 7 Dorsum: 2	Glabella: 9 Nasolabial fold: 2 Dorsum: 5	Not significant
No. of injections in study	22	13	Not significant

Annual incidence of cosmetic 20,000; 90,000 not tested; ISAPS survey on injections aesthetic procedures.
Abbreviations: ISAPS, International Society of Aesthetic Plastic Surgery; SD, standard deviation.
From Thomas WW, Bucky L, Friedman O. Injectables in the nose: facts and controversies. Facial Plast Surg Clin North Am. 2016;24(3):387; with permission.

In arterial accidents, in which skin blanching is not resolving in minutes, some authors suggest that repositioning the patient to Trendelenburg using vasodilator pastes such as nitroglycerine, and hand rubbing the area could be beneficial.[53]

Fat hypertrophy is usually associated with extreme weight gain and may cause some deformities like contour distortion or irregularities. However, the good point is that this kind of changes will disappear with wight loss.[60]

FILLERS

The most important characteristics of HA is that HA can be resolved by hyaluronidase (HYAL). This quality let us to address many major problems associated with fillers, including high-volume injection or injections in inappropriate places like too superficially or too deep injections, or even injecting in the vessels.[190]

Hyaluronidase is an enzyme that resolves both simple and cross-linked HA. The source of hyaluronidase varies. In general, there are 3 different sources: the first is an animal resource, especially mammalian; the second is from bacteria; and third are from some species like crustaceans, leeches, and parasites.[120]

There are no specific guidelines for using HYAL, and in previous articles, various approaches to using HYAL have been mentioned. However, titration until resolving the HA seems to be a point of agreement. Some authors are advocates of using 150 IU in the beginning and using as high as 1500 IU for vascular congestions.[190] To dilute HYAL, some authors suggest normal saline, some would suggest lidocaine, or many other solvents, but the most important point is the pH, which must not be compromised because of some unpredictable changes to its efficacy.[190] After injecting HYAL, mechanical massage is applied on the area for effective influence and covering of HA by HYAL.[190]

The reaction of immune system is one of the complications that needs to be considered. In the past, because of the animal source of the HYAL, there were more reports of allergy, especially to bovine resources. Anaphylactic allergy can occur in persons who have had history of insect bites or stings owing to resources of HYAL in their stings.[190] Another complication is the Tyndall effect. This phenomenon occurs when filler is injected too superficially, which could lead to a bluish color immediately under the superficial layer. This complication is addressed by HYAL as well, and subsequent massage or using a small needle incision and mechanical removal.[145,191–193]

Nodules and lumps are another complication one may encounter during injection and they are due to the injection of large amount of material to a specific area. Using small stab incisions or needles for aspiration, or occasionally using HYAL, are suggested treatments. When using HYAL, a history of establishing the nodules and differentiation of infected HA is important.[194–200]

Infection is another rare complication may happen after injecting any materials or implants.[201] Infection can occur because of bacteria, viruses, or fungal sources, such as *Candida*.[190] generally, it seems that infection with herpes simplex virus is the most common infection encountered during filler injection. Histories of having multiple herpes simplex infections suggest using antiviral agents.[190] Bacterial infection is usually associated with technical procedures. For example, a single area infection may occur owing to skin bacterial infection, or in case of multiple infections, it may be a result of syringe contaminations. If the source of infection is not immediately apparent, using both antivirals and antibiotics is recommended. In immunocompromised persons or those with infections resistant to treatment, consider fungal infections must be considered.[202] There is no single accepted procedure for skin preparation, but preparation with 2% chlorhexidine gluconate solute in 70% alcohol is recommended by some authors.[190]

Vascular accident is a serious complication. Some injectable materials cause worse complications when they are injected to vascular system because they trigger inflammatory and clotting reactions; these entities include fat and collagen.[203–209] Most HA do not incite inflammatory processes and the only effect is the obstructive action. In some cases, it could cause heparin-like behaviors.[210,211] Vascular obstruction is also called embolia cutis medicamentosa, Nicolau syndrome, or Freudenthal–Nicolau syndrome.

Vascular injection could cause problematic events, some of which depend on artery obstruction or vein obstruction. In either case, hypoxia owing to obstruction is the cause. The changes range from blanching to bluish skin color and necrosis of the affected area in a few minutes to a few days.[31] In severe cases, there are reports of blindness, stroke, and extensive tissue necrosis.[36,210–224]

Pain usually is the first sign of vascular obstruction. In patients who are given anesthetic agents, this symptom is absent. Blanching is often accompanied by pain, and often happens immediately after injection in an artery, although this is not pathognomonic. Again, for patients who received anesthetic agents with epinephrine, it may be a common finding. The greatest effect of epinephrine happens at approximately 7 minutes, but, in arterial obstruction, it lasts more than 7 minutes and happens immediately after injection. A reliable finding is a skin pattern that is called livedo reticularis, a reaction to cold, that also occurs in vascular obstruction after hypoxic color changes of the skin to bluish or purple owing to a decrease of oxygen in the tissue. The other sign is slow capillary refill. By finger pressure on the skin, 1 to 2 seconds is assumed as a normal time for capillary refill. In arterial obstruction, this procedure takes more time than usual. In venous obstruction,

very fast capillary refill happens in a bluish skin. In the presence of cold or epinephrine injection, this sign is not reliable. A bluish and gray color to the skin is the next phase, as a result of deoxygenation. If this condition persists, the skin and all the infarcted portion of tissue, which was bleeding by that specific artery, will be necrotic. In the end, healing will occur by secondary intention in a limited area, whereas in the extended area, reconstruction of the wound requires skin flaps.[36]

There are some reports of blindness and stroke owing to filler or fat injection to the face, because of the anastomoses of external carotid and internal carotid arteries. This can happen to ipsilateral eye or contralateral eye. In similar cases of complete or partial vision loss, the patient must immediately be referred to an ophthalmologist for fundoscopy and further treatment. Overall, in an artery obstruction that leads to skin or tissue ischemia, time plays an important role, so the potential crisis management should be considered.[190]

With the attention to some points we could prevent artery accidents:

1. The volume of material that is injected in a specific area in each time. It is recommended that it should not be more than 0.1 mL.
2. Recognition of the injecting area anatomy! The practitioner should have a good understanding of danger zones like angular artery, or glabella or nasolabial fold anatomy. In addition, considering aspiration before injecting the material, injecting while withdrawing the needle back and avoiding high pressure.
3. Using a sharp and small gauge needle exposes the patient to a high risk of artery accident, especially in patients with scar tissue, because they are prone to the possibility of needle entering to an immovable and steady artery lying in the area. So, it is recommended that practitioners use a blunt cannula to decrease the risk of artery injection.

CLINICS CARE POINTS

- Proper patient selection may be the backbone of the non surgical rhinoplasty.
- Inform the patient about the risks and benefits of the procedure.
- Use the correct method of fat preparation and if possible use stem cells and new methods of preparation.
- Use suitable processing and injection equipment.
- Inject a little more fat than needed.
- Follow the patient carefully and if he/she shows critical symptoms, act urgently.

- Inform the patient about the possibility of the need to repeat the procedure.
- Use a standard filler.

ACKNOWLEDGEMENT

The authors thank Craniomaxillofacial Research Center, Shariatic Hospital, Tehran university of Medical Sciences, Tehran, Iran.

DISCLOSURE

The authors have nothing to disclose.

REFERENCES

1. Monreal J. Fat grafting to the nose: personal experience with 36 patients. Aesthet Plast Surg 2011; 35(5):916.
2. Jasin ME. Nonsurgical rhinoplasty using dermal fillers. Facial Plast Surg Clin 2013;21(2):241–52.
3. Baptista C, Nguyen PSA, Desouches C, et al. Correction of sequelae of rhinoplasty by lipofilling. J Plast Reconstr Aesthet Surg 2013;66(6):805–11.
4. Waite PD. Avoiding revision rhinoplasty. Oral Maxill Surg Clin North America 2011;23(1):93–100.
5. Guerrerosantos J. Temporoparietal free fascia grafts in rhinoplasty. Plast Reconstr Surg 1984; 74(4):465–75.
6. Nakakita N, Sezaki K, Yamazaki Y, et al. Augmentation rhinoplasty using an L-shaped auricular cartilage framework combined with dermal fat graft for cleft lip nose. Aesthet Plast Surg 1999;23(2): 107–12.
7. Toriumi DM. Skeletal modifications in rhinoplasty. Facial Plast Surg Clin North Am 2000;8:413–31.
8. Baker TM, Courtiss EH. Temporalis fascia grafts in open secondary rhinoplasty. Plast Reconstr Surg 1994;93(4):802–10.
9. Daniel RK, Calvert JW. Diced cartilage grafts in rhinoplasty surgery. Plast Reconstr Surg 2004;113(7): 2156–71.
10. Khurana D, Sherris DA. Grafting materials for augmentation septorhinoplasty. Curr Opin Otolaryngol Head Neck Surg 1999;7(4):210.
11. Toriumi DM. Autogenous grafts are worth the extra time. Arch Otolaryngol Head Neck Surg 2000; 126(4):562–4.
12. Watson D, Toriumi DM. Injertos estructurales en rinoplastia secundaria. In: Gunter JP, Rohrich RJ, Adams WP Jr, editors. Rinoplastia de Dallas: Cirugía nasal por los maestros. 1st edition. St Louis (MO): AMOLCA; 2003. p. 691–709.
13. Bracaglia R, Fortunato R, Gentileschi S. Secondary rhinoplasty. Aesthet Plast Surg 2005;29(4):230–9.
14. Cárdenas JC, Carvajal J. Refinement of rhinoplasty with lipoinjection. Aesthet Plast Surg 2007;31(5): 501–5.
15. Lee MR, Unger JG, Rohrich RJ. Management of the nasal dorsum in rhinoplasty: a systematic review of the literature regarding technique, outcomes, and complications. Plast Reconstr Surg 2011;128(5): 538e–50e.
16. Wee JH, Park MH, Oh S, et al. Complications associated with autologous rib cartilage use in rhinoplasty: a meta-analysis. JAMA Facial Plast Surg 2015;17(1):49–55.
17. Peled ZM, Warren AG, Johnston P, et al. The use of alloplastic materials in rhinoplasty surgery: a meta-analysis. Plast Reconstr Surg 2008;121(3): 85e–92e.
18. Kao WP, Lin YN, Lin TY, et al. Microautologous fat transplantation for primary augmentation rhinoplasty: long-term monitoring of 198 Asian patients. Aesthet Surg J 2016;36(6):648–56.
19. Stein A. Paraffin-injektionen. Therorie und Praxis: Eine Zusammenfassende Darstellung Ihrer Verwendung in Allen Spezialfachern Der Medizin (German) Paperback. 1904;79e114.
20. Thomas WW, Bucky L, Friedman O. Injectables in the nose: facts and controversies. Facial Plast Surg Clin 2016;24(3):379–89.
21. Kornstein AN, Nikfarjam JS. Fat grafting to the forehead/glabella/radix complex and pyriform aperture: aesthetic and anti-aging implications. Plast Reconstr Surg Glob Open 2015;3(8):e500.
22. Sheen JH, Sheen AP. Aesthetic rhinoplasty, vol. 1. : Mosby Incorporated; 1987.
23. McKinney P, Sweis I. A clinical definition of an ideal nasal radix. Plast Reconstr Surg 2002;109(4):1416–8.
24. Constantian MB. An alternate strategy for reducing the large nasal base. Plast Reconstr Surg 1989; 83(1):41–52.
25. Fontana AM, Muti E. Surgery of the naso-frontal angle. Aesthet Plast Surg 1996;20(4):319–22.
26. Pessa JE, Desvigne LD, Zadoo VP. The effect of skeletal remodeling on the nasal profile: considerations for rhinoplasty in the older patient. Aesthet Plast Surg 1999;23(4):239–42.
27. Shaw RB Jr, Katzel EB, Koltz PF, et al. Aging of the facial skeleton: aesthetic implications and rejuvenation strategies. Plast Reconstr Surg 2011; 127(1):374–83.
28. Haffner CL, Pessa JE, Zadoo VP, et al. A technique for three-dimensional cephalometric analysis as an aid in evaluating changes in the craniofacial skeleton. Angle Orthodontist 1999; 69(4):345–8.
29. Hoffmann C, Schuller-Petrovic S, Soyer HP, et al. Adverse reactions after cosmetic lip augmentation with permanent biologically inert implant materials. J Am Acad Dermatol 1999;40(1):100–2.
30. Erol OO. Microfat grafting in nasal surgery. Aesthet Surg J 2014;34(5):671–86.

31. Fitzpatrick TB, Elsen AZ, Wolff K, et al. Dermatology in general medicine. 4th edition. New York: McGraw; 1993.

32. Braverman IM, Keh-Yen A. Ultrastructure of the human dermal microcirculation. IV. Valve-containing collecting veins at the dermal–subcutaneous junction. J Invest Dermatol 1983;81(5):438–42.

33. Braverman IM, Keh-Yen A. Ultrastructure of the human dermal microcirculation. III. The vessels in the mid-and lower dermis and subcutaneous fat. J Invest Dermatol 1981;77(3):297–304.

34. Braverman IM, Yen A. Ultrastructure of the capillary loops in the dermal papillae of psoriasis. J Invest Dermatol 1977;68(1):53–60.

35. Yen A, Braverman IM. Ultrastructure of the human dermal microcirculation: the horizontal plexus of the papillary dermis. J Invest Dermatol 1976;66(3):131–42.

36. DeLorenzi C. Complications of injectable fillers, part 2: vascular complications. Aesthet Surg J 2014;34(4):584–600.

37. Braverman IM, Keh A, Goldminz D. Correlation of laser Doppler wave patterns with underlying microvascular anatomy. J Invest Dermatol 1990;95(3):283–6.

38. Duval A, Pouchot J. Livedo: de la physiopathologie au diagnostic. La Revue de médecine interne 2008;29(5):380–92.

39. Billings E Jr, May JW Jr. Historical review and present status of free fat graft autotransplantation in plastic and reconstructive surgery. Plast Reconstr Surg 1989;83(2):368–81.

40. Simonacci F, Bertozzi N, Grieco MP, et al. Procedure, applications, and outcomes of autologous fat grafting. Ann Med Surg 2017;20:49–60.

41. Bruning P. Contribution a l'etude des greffes adipeuses. Bull Acad R Med Belg 1919;28:440.

42. Peer LA. Loss of weight and volume in human fat grafts: with postulation of a "cell survival theory". Plast Reconstr Surg 1950;5(3):217–30.

43. Rivkin A. A prospective study of non-surgical primary rhinoplasty using a polymethylmethacrylate injectable implant. Dermatol Surg 2014;40(3):305–13.

44. Khawaja HA, Hernández-Pérez E. Fat transfer review: controversies, complications, their prevention, and treatment. Int J Cosmet Surg Aesthet Dermatol 2002;4(2):131–8.

45. Coleman SR. Structural fat grafting. Aesthet Surg J 1998;18(5):386–8.

46. Lin TM, Lin SD, Lai CS. (2007, May). The treatment of nasolabial fold with free fat graft: preliminary concept of Micro-Autologous Fat Transplantation (MAFT). In 2nd academic congress of Taiwan Cosmetic Association Taipei, Taiwan.

47. Chou CK, Lin TM, Chou C. Influential factors in autologous fat transplantation—focusing on the lumen size of injection needle and the injecting volume. J IPRAS 2013;9:25–7.

48. Micro-Autologous Fat Transplantation (MAFT) for the Correction of Sunken Temporal Fossa-Long Term Follow up. 2012.

49. Lin TM, Lin TY, Chou CK, et al. Application of micro-autologous fat transplantation in the correction of sunken upper eyelid. Plast Reconstr Surg Glob Open 2014;2(11):e259.

50. Lin TM, Lin TY, Huang YH, Hsieh TY, Chou CK, Takahashi H,, Lin SD. Fat grafting for recontouring sunken upper eyelids with multiple folds in Asians—novel mechanism for neoformation of double eyelid crease. Ann Plast Surg 2016;76(4):371–5.

51. Lin TM. Total Facial Rejuvenation with Micro-Autologous Fat Transplantation (MAFT). In: Pu LLQ, Chen YR, Li QF, et al, editors. Aesthetic plastic surgery in Asians: principles and techniques. 1st edition. St Louis (MO): CRC Press; 2015. p. 127–46.

52. Alexander RW. Liposculpture in the superficial plane: closed syringe system for improvements in fat removal and free fat transfer. Am J Cosmet Surg 1994;11(2):127–34.

53. Marwah M, Kulkarni A, Godse K, et al. Fat ful'fill'ment: a review of autologous fat grafting. J Cutan Aesthet Surg 2013;6(3):132.

54. Venkataram J. Tumescent liposuction: a review. J Cutan Aesthet Surg 2008;1(2):49.

55. Gir P, Brown SA, Oni G, et al. Fat grafting: evidence-based review on autologous fat harvesting, processing, reinjection, and storage. Plast Reconstr Surg 2012;130(1):249–58.

56. Pu LL, Cui X, Fink BF, et al. Long-term preservation of adipose aspirates after conventional lipoplasty. Aesthet Surg J 2004;24(6):536–41.

57. Nguyen A, Pasyk KA, Bouvier TN, et al. Comparative study of survival of autologous adipose tissue taken and transplanted by different techniques. Plast Reconstr Surg 1990;85(3):378–86.

58. Coleman SR. Facial recontouring with lipostructure. Clin Plast Surg 1997;24(2):347–67.

59. Bersou Júnior A. Lipoenxertia: técnica expansiva. Rev Bras Cir Plást 2008;23(2):89–97.

60. Amarante M. Analysis of structured fat grafting for redefining facial contours. Revista Brasileira de Cirurgia Plástica 2001;28(1):49–54.

61. Katz AJ, Llull R, Hedrick MH, et al. Emerging approaches to the tissue engineering of fat. Clin Plast Surg 1999;26(4):587–603.

62. Raposio E, Guida C, Baldelli I, et al. Characterization and induction of human preadipocytes. Toxicol In Vitro 2007;21:330e334.

63. Raposio E, Guida C, Coradeghini R, et al. In vitro polydeoxyribonucleotide effects on human preadipocytes. Cell Prolif 2008;41:739e754.

64. Raposio E, Bertozzi N, Bonomini S, et al. Adipose-derived stem cells added to platelet-rich plasma for chronic skin ulcer therapy. Wounds 2016;28:126e131.

65. Higuchi A, Chuang CW, Ling QD, Huang SC, Wang LM, Chen H,, Hsu ST. Differentiation ability of adipose-derived stem cells separated from adipose tissue by a membrane filtration method. J Membr Sci 2011;366(1–2):286–94.

66. Salibian AA, Widgerow AD, Abrouk M, et al. Stem cells in plastic surgery: a review of current clinical and translational applications. Arch Plast Surg 2013;40(6):666.

67. Caruana G, Bertozzi N, Boschi E, et al. Role of adipose-derived stem cells in chronic cutaneous wound healing. Ann Ital Chir 2015;86(1):1–4.

68. Coleman SR. Long-term survival of fat transplants: controlled demonstrations. Aesthet Plast Surg 1995;19(5):421–5.

69. Leong DT, Hutmacher DW, Chew FT, et al. Viability and adipogenic potential of human adipose tissue processed cell population obtained from pump-assisted and syringe-assisted liposuction. J Dermatol Sci 2005;37(3):169–76.

70. Tremolada C, Palmieri G, Ricordi C. Adipocyte transplantation and stem cells: plastic surgery meets regenerative medicine. Cell Transplant 2010;19(10):1217–23.

71. Ferraro GA, De Francesco F, Tirino V, et al. Effects of a new centrifugation method on adipose cell viability for autologous fat grafting. Aesthet Plast Surg 2011;35(3):341–8.

72. Kakagia D, Pallua N. Autologous fat grafting: in search of the optimal technique. Surg innovation 2014;21(3):327–36.

73. Fagrell D, Eneström S, Berggren A, et al. Fat cylinder transplantation: an experimental comparative study of three different kinds of fat transplants. Plast Reconstr Surg 1996;98(1):90–6.

74. Qin W, Xu Y, Liu X, et al. Experimental and primary clinical research of core fat graft. Zhongguo Xiu Fu Chong Jian Wai Ke Za Zhi 2012;26(5):576–82.

75. Pu LL, Cui X, Fink BF, et al. The viability of fatty tissues within adipose aspirates after conventional liposuction: a comprehensive study. Ann Plast Surg 2005;54(3):288–92.

76. Pu LL, Coleman SR, Cui X, et al. Autologous fat grafts harvested and refined by the Coleman technique: a comparative study. Plast Reconstr Surg 2008;122(3):932–7.

77. Özsoy Z, Kul Z, Bilir A. The role of cannula diameter in improved adipocyte viability: a quantitative analysis. Aesthet Surg J 2006;26(3):287–9.

78. Campbell GL, Laudenslager N, Newman J. The effect of mechanical stress on adipocyte morphology and metabolism. Am J Cosmet Surg 1987;4(2):89–94.

79. Erdim M, Tezel E, Numanoglu A, et al. The effects of the size of liposuction cannula on adipocyte survival and the optimum temperature for fat graft storage: an experimental study. J Plast Reconstr Aesthet Surg 2009;62(9):1210–4.

80. Coleman SR. Structural fat grafting: more than a permanent filler. Plast Reconstr Surg 2006;118(3S):108S–20S.

81. Crawford JL, Hubbard BA, Colbert SH, et al. Fine tuning lipoaspirate viability for fat grafting. Plast Reconstr Surg 2010;126(4):1342–8.

82. Hamza A, Lohsiriwat V, Rietjens M. Lipofilling in breast cancer surgery. Gland Surg 2013;2(1):7.

83. Klein JA. Tumescent technique for local anesthesia improves safety in large-volume lipoauction. Plast Reconstr Surg 1993;92:1085.

84. Kasem A, Wazir U, Headon H, et al. Breast lipofilling: a review of current practice. Arch Plast Surg 2015;42(2):126.

85. Botti G, Pascali M, Botti C, et al. A clinical trial in facial fat grafting: filtered and washed versus centrifuged fat. Plast Reconstr Surg 2011;127(6):2464–73.

86. Khater R, Atanassova P, Anastassov Y, et al. Clinical and experimental study of autologous fat grafting after processing by centrifugation and serum lavage. Aesthet Plast Surg 2009;33:37e43.

87. Wilson A, Butler PE, Seifalian AM. Adipose-derived stem cells for clinical applications: a review. Cell Prolif 2011;44(1):86–98.

88. Tuin AJ, Domerchie PN, Schepers RH, et al. What is the current optimal fat grafting processing technique? A systematic review. J Craniomaxillofac Surg 2016;44:45e55.

89. Condé-Green A, de Amorim NFG, Pitanguy I. Influence of decantation, washing and centrifugation on adipocyte and mesenchymal stem cell content of aspirated adipose tissue: a comparative study. J Plast Reconstr Aesthet Surg 2010;63(8):1375–81.

90. Mojallal A, Foyatier JL. The effect of different factors on the survival of transplanted adipocytes. Ann Chir Plast Esthet 2004;49(5):426–36.

91. Carpaneda CA, Ribeiro MT. Percentage of graft viability versus injected volume in adipose autotransplants. Aesthet Plast Surg 1994;18(1):17–9.

92. Carraway J. Autologous fat grafting: is it a useful procedure? Aesthet Surg J 1996;16(1):13–5.

93. Guerrerosantos J, Haidar F, Paillet JC. Aesthetic facial contour augmentation with microlipofilling. Aesthet Surg J 2003;23(4):239–47.

94. Karacaoglu E, Kizilkaya E, Cermik H, et al. The role of recipient sites in fat-graft survival: experimental study. Ann Plast Surg 2005;55(1):63–8.

95. Kern S, Eichler H, Stoeve J, et al. Comparative analysis of mesenchymal stem cells from bone

marrow, umbilical cord blood, or adipose tissue. Stem cells 2006;24(5):1294–301.

96. Lee RH, Kim B, Choi I, Kim H, Choi HS, Suh K,, Jung JS. Characterization and expression analysis of mesenchymal stem cells from human bone marrow and adipose tissue. Cell Physiol Biochem 2004;14(4–6):311–24.

97. Coradeghini R, Guida C, Scanarotti C, et al. A comparative study of proliferation and hepatic differentiation of human adipose-derived stem cells. Cells Tissues Organs 2010;191:466e477.

98. Aluigi MG, Coradeghini R, Guida C, Scanarotti C, Bassi AM, Falugi C,, Raposio E. Pre-adipocytes commitment to neurogenesis 1: preliminary localisation of cholinergic molecules. Cell Biol Int 2009;33(5):594–601.

99. Scanarotti C, Bassi AM, Catalano M, et al. Neurogenic-committed human pre-adipocytes express CYP1A isoforms. Chem Biol Interact 2010;184(3):474–83.

100. Raposio E, Caruana G, Petrella M, et al. A standardized method of isolating adipose-derived stem cells for clinical applications. Ann Plast Surg 2016;76(1):124–6.

101. Raposio E, Caruana G, Bonomini S, et al. A novel and effective strategy for the isolation of adipose-derived stem cells: minimally manipulated adipose-derived stem cells for more rapid and safe stem cell therapy. Plast Reconstr Surg 2014; 133(6):1406–9.

102. Matsumoto D, Sato K, Gonda K, Takaki Y, Shigeura T, Sato T,, Yoshimura K. Cell-assisted lipotransfer: supportive use of human adipose-derived cells for soft tissue augmentation with lipoinjection. Tissue Eng 2006;12(12):3375–82.

103. Zuk PA, Zhu MIN, Mizuno H, et al. Multilineage cells from human adipose tissue: implications for cell-based therapies. Tissue Eng 2001;7(2):211–28.

104. Padoin AV, Braga-Silva J, Martins P, et al. Sources of processed lipoaspirate cells: influence of donor site on cell concentration. Plast Reconstr Surg 2008;122:614–8.

105. Ashjian PH, De Ugarte DA, Katz AJ, et al. Lipoplasty: from body contouring to tissue engineering. Aesthet Surg J 2002;22(2):121–7.

106. Kokai LE, Rubin JP, Marra KG. The potential of adipose-derived adult stem cells as a source of neuronal progenitor cells. Plast Reconstr Surg 2005;116(5):1453–60.

107. Rubin JP, Agha-Mohammadi S. Mesenchymal stem cells: aesthetic applications. Aesthet Surg J 2003; 23(6):504–6.

108. di Summa PG, Kingham PJ, Raffoul W, et al. Adipose-derived stem cells enhance peripheral nerve regeneration. J Plast Reconstr Aesthet Surg 2010; 63(9):1544–52.

109. Guo A, Owens WA, Coady M, et al. An in vivo mouse model of human skin replacement for wound healing and cell therapy studies. J Plast Reconstr Aesthet Surg 2012;65(8):1129–31.

110. Itoi Y, Takatori M, Hyakusoku H, et al. Comparison of readily available scaffolds for adipose tissue engineering using adipose-derived stem cells. J Plast Reconstr Aesthet Surg 2010;63(5):858–64.

111. Zografou A, Tsigris C, Papadopoulos O, et al. Improvement of skin-graft survival after autologous transplantation of adipose-derived stem cells in rats. J Plast Reconstr Aesthet Surg 2011;64(12): 1647–56.

112. Sterodimas A, de Faria J, Nicaretta B, et al. Tissue engineering with adipose-derived stem cells (ADSCs): current and future applications. J Plast Reconstr Aesthet Surg 2010;63(11):1886–92.

113. Lin S, Hsiao YC, Huang JJ, et al. Minimal invasive rhinoplasty: fat injection for nasal dorsum contouring. Ann Plast Surg 2017;78(3):S117–23.

114. Del Vecchio D, Rohrich RJ. A classification of clinical fat grafting: different problems, different solutions. Plast Reconstr Surg 2012;130(3): 511–22.

115. Umeno H, Chitose S, Sato K, et al. Comparative study of framework surgery and fat injection laryngoplasty. The J Laryngol Otology 2009;123(S31): 35–41.

116. Tamura E, Fukuda H, Tabata Y, et al. Use of the buccal fad pad for vocal cord augmentation. Acta Otolaryngol 2008;128(2):219–24.

117. Gabrick K, Walker M, Timberlake A, et al. The effect of autologous fat grafting on edema and ecchymoses in primary open rhinoplasty. Aesthet Surg J 2020;40(4):359–66.

118. Webster RC, Hamdan US, Gaunt JM, et al. Rhinoplastic revisions with injectable silicone. Arch Otolaryngol Head Neck Surg 1986;112(3):269–76.

119. Meyer K, Palmer JW. The polysaccharide of the vitreous humor. J Biol Chem 1934;107(3):629–34.

120. Garg HG, Hales CA, editors. Chemistry and biology of hyaluronan. Elsevier; 2004.

121. Nusgens BV. April). Hyaluronic acid and extracellular matrix: a primitive molecule? Ann Dermatol Vénéréol 2010;137:S3–8.

122. Ascher B, Cerceau M, Baspeyras M, et al. Soft tissue filling with hyaluronic acid. Ann Chir Plast Esthet 2004;49(5):465–85.

123. Fraser JRE, Laurent TC, Laurent UBG. Hyaluronan: its nature, distribution, functions and turnover. J Intern Med 1997;242(1):27–33.

124. Fraser JR, Dahl LB, Kimpton WG, et al. Elimination and subsequent metabolism of circulating hyaluronic acid in the fetus. J Dev Physiol 1989;11(4): 235–42.

125. Fraser JR, Laurent TC. January). Turnover and metabolism of hyaluronan. Ciba Found Symp 1989;143(No. 1):41–53.

126. Laurent TC. Biochemistry of hyaluronan. Acta Otolaryngol 1987;104(sup442):7–24.

127. Laurent TC, Dahl IMS, Dahl LB, et al. The catabolic fate of hyaluronic acid. Connect Tissue Res 1986; 15(1–2):33–41.

128. Fraser JRE, Laurent TC, Engström-Laurent A, et al. Elimination of hyaluronic acid from the blood stream in the human. Clin Exp Pharmacol Physiol 1984;11(1):17–25.

129. Tezel A, Fredrickson GH. The science of hyaluronic acid dermal fillers. J Cosmet Laser Ther 2008; 10(1):35–42.

130. Lowe NJ, Maxwell CA, Patnaik R. Adverse reactions to dermal fillers. Dermatol Surg 2005;31: 1626–33.

131. Curcio NM, Parish LC. Injectable fillers: an American perspective. Giornale italiano di dermatologia e venereologia: organo ufficiale. Societa italiana di dermatologia e sifilografia 2009; 144(3):271–9.

132. Ellis DA, Segall L. Review of Non–FDA-Approved Fillers. Facial Plast Surg Clin North Am 2007; 15(2):239–46.

133. Kontis TC, Rivkin A. The history of injectable facial fillers. Facial Plast Surg 2009;25(02):067–72.

134. Wesley NO, Dover JS. The filler revolution: a six-year retrospective. J Drugs Dermatol 2009;8(10): 903–7.

135. Rivkin A. New fillers under consideration: what is the future of injectable aesthetics? Facial Plast Surg 2009;25(02):120–3.

136. Goldberg DJ. Breakthroughs in US dermal fillers for facial soft-tissue augmentation. J Cosmet Laser Ther 2009;11(4):240–7.

137. Sundaram H, Voigts B, Beer K, et al. Comparison of the rheological properties of viscosity and elasticity in two categories of soft tissue fillers: calcium hydroxylapatite and hyaluronic acid. Dermatol Surg 2010;36:1859–65.

138. Humphrey CD, Arkins JP, Dayan SH. Soft tissue fillers in the nose. Aesthet Surg J 2009;29(6): 477–84.

139. Nyte CP. Spreader graft injection with calcium hydroxylapatite: a nonsurgical technique for internal nasal valve collapse. The Laryngoscope 2006;116(7):1291–2.

140. Graivier MH, Bass LS, Busso M, et al. Calcium hydroxylapatite (Radiesse) for correction of the mid-and lower face: consensus recommendations. Plast Reconstr Surg 2007;120(6S):55S–66S.

141. Smith KC. Reversible vs. nonreversible fillers in facial aesthetics: concerns and considerations. Dermatol Online J 2008;14(8):3.

142. Park TH, Seo SW, Kim JK, et al. Clinical experience with hyaluronic acid-filler complications. J Plast Reconstr Aesthet Surg 2011;64(7):892–6.

143. Menon H, Thomas M, D'silva J. Low dose of Hyaluronidase to treat over correction by HA filler–A Case Report. J Plast Reconstr Aesthet Surg 2010; 63(4):e416–7.

144. Rzany B, Becker-Wegerich P, Bachmann F, et al. Hyaluronidase in the correction of hyaluronic acid-based fillers: a review and a recommendation for use. J Cosmet Dermatol 2009;8(4):317–23.

145. Hirsch RJ, Brody HJ, Carruthers JD. Hyaluronidase in the office: a necessity for every dermasurgeon that injects hyaluronic acid. J Cosmet Laser Ther 2007;9(3):182–5.

146. Pierre A, Levy PM. Hyaluronidase offers an efficacious treatment for inaesthetic hyaluronic acid overcorrection. J Cosmet Dermatol 2007;6(3): 159–62.

147. Brody HJ. Use of hyaluronidase in the treatment of granulomatous hyaluronic acid reactions or unwanted hyaluronic acid misplacement. Dermatol Surg 2005;31(8):893–7.

148. Lambros V. The use of hyaluronidase to reverse the effects of hyaluronic acid filler. Plast Reconstr Surg 2004;114(1):277.

149. Soparkar CN, Patrinely JR, Tschen J. Erasing restylane. Ophthalmic Plast Reconstr Surg 2004;20(4): 317–8.

150. Knapp TR, Vistnes LM. The augmentation of soft tissue with injectable collagen. Clin Plast Surg 1985;12:221–5.

151. Han SK, Shin SH, Kang HJ, et al. Augmentation rhinoplasty using injectable tissue-engineered soft tissue. Ann Plast Surg 2006;56:251–5.

152. Beer KR. Nasal reconstruction using 20mg/mL cross-linked hyaluronic acid. J Drugs Dermatol 2006;5:465–6.

153. Becker H. Nasal augmentation with calcium hydroxylapatite in a carrier-based gel. Plast Reconstr Surg 2008;121:2142–7.

154. Rokhsar C, Ciocon DH. Nonsurgical rhinoplasty: an evaluation of injectable calcium hydroxylapatite filler for nasal contouring. Dermatol Surg 2008;4: 944–6.

155. de Lacerda BA, Zancanaro P. Filler rhinoplasty. Dermatol Surg 2007;3:S207–12.

156. Cassuto D. The use of dermicol-P35 dermal filler for nonsurgical rhinoplasty. Aesthet Surg J 2009; 29:522–4.

157. Siclovan HR, Jomah JA. Injectable calcium hydroxylapatite for correction of nasal bridge deformities. Aesthetic Plast Surg 2009;33:544–8.

158. Rivkin A, Soliemanzadeh P. Nonsurgical rhinoplastywith calcium hydroxylapatite (Radiesse®). Cosmet Dermatol 2009;12:619–24.

159. Bray D, Hopkins C, Roberts DN. Injection rhinoplasty: non-surgical nasal augmentation and correction of post-rhinoplasty contour asymmetries with hyaluronic acid: how we do it. Clin Otolaryngol 2010;35:220–37.

160. Dayan SH, Kempiners JJ. Treatment of the lower third of the nose and dynamic nasal tip ptosis with Botox. Plast Reconstr Surg 2005;115:1784–5.

161. Kim P, Ahn JT. Structured nonsurgical Asian rhinoplasty. Aesthetic Plast Surg 2012;36:698–703.

162. Coleman SR, Saboeiro AP. Fat grafting to the breast revisited: safety and efficacy. Plast Reconstr Surg 2007;119(3):775–85.

163. Gutowski KA, Force AFGT. Current applications and safety of autologous fat grafts: a report of the ASPS fat graft task force. Plast Reconstr Surg 2009;124(1):272–80.

164. Delay E, Garson S, Tousson G, et al. Fat injection to the breast: technique, results, and indications based on 880 procedures over 10 years. Aesthet Surg J 2009;29(5):360–76.

165. Illouz YG, Sterodimas A. Autologous fat transplantation to the breast: a personal technique with 25 years of experience. Aesthet Plast Surg 2009;33(5):706–15.

166. Chan CW, McCulley SJ, Macmillan RD. Autologous fat transfer–a review of the literature with a focus on breast cancer surgery. J Plast Reconstr Aesthet Surg 2008;61(12):1438–48.

167. Agha RA, Fowler AJ, Herlin C, et al. Use of autologous fat grafting for breast reconstruction: a systematic review with meta-analysis of oncological outcomes. J Plast Reconstr Aesthet Surg 2015;68(2):143–61.

168. Butterwick KJ. Rejuvenation of the aging hand. Dermatol Clin 2005;23(3):515–27.

169. Fournier PF. Fat transfer to the hand for rejuvenation. In: Shiffman MA, editor. Autologous fat transfer. Berlin: Springer; 2010. p. 273–80.

170. Vara AD, Miki RA, Alfonso DT, et al. Hand fat grafting complicated by abscess: a case of a bilateral hand abscess from bilateral hand fat grafting. Hand 2013;8(3):348–51.

171. Miller JJ, Popp JC. Fat hypertrophy after autologous fat transfer. Ophthalmic Plast Reconstr Surg 2002;18(3):228–31.

172. Teimourian B, Adham MN. Rejuvenation of the hand: fat injection combined with TCA peel. Aesthet Surg J 2000;20(1):70–1.

173. Ersek RA. Transplantation of purified autologous fat: a 3-year follow-up is disappointing. Plast Reconstr Surg 1991;87(2):219–27.

174. Choi M, Small K, Levovitz C, et al. The volumetric analysis of fat graft survival in breast reconstruction. Plast Reconstr Surg 2013;131(2):185–91.

175. Mojallal A, Shipkov C, Braye F, et al. Influence of the recipient site on the outcomes of fat grafting in facial reconstructive surgery. Plast Reconstr Surg 2009;124(2):471–83.

176. Zhu M, Cohen SR, Hicok KC, Shanahan RK, Strem BM, Johnson CY,, Fraser JK. Comparison of three different fat graft preparation methods: gravity separation, centrifugation, and simultaneous washing with filtration in a closed system. Plast Reconstr Surg 2013;131(4):873–80.

177. Asilian A, Siadat AH, Iraji R. Comparison of fat maintenance in the face with centrifuge versus filtered and washed fat. J Res Med Sci 2014;19(6):556.

178. Hoang D, Orgel MI, Kulber DA. Hand rejuvenation: a comprehensive review of fat grafting. J Hand Surg 2016;41(5):639–44.

179. Obagi S. Autologous fat augmentation and periorbital laser resurfacing complicated by abscess formation. Am J Cosmet Surg 2003;20(3):155–7.

180. Boureaux E, Chaput B, Bannani S, et al. Eyelid fat grafting: indications, operative technique and complications; a systematic review. J Craniomaxillofac Surg 2016;44:374e380.

181. Park SH, Sun HJ, Choi KS. Sudden unilateral visual loss after autologous fat injection into the nasolabial fold. Clin Ophthalmol 2008;2:679e683.

182. Dreizen NG, Framm L. Sudden unilateral visual loss after autologous fat injection into the glabellar area. Am J Ophthalmol 1989;107:85–7.

183. Feinendegen DL, Baumgartner RW, Schroth G, et al. Middle cerebral artery occlusion and ocular fat embolism after autologous fat injection in the face. J Neurol 1998;1(245):53–4.

184. Yoon SS, Chang DI, Chung KC. Acute fatal stroke immediately following autologous fat injection into the face. Neurology 2003;61(8):1151–2.

185. Park KH, Kim YK, Woo SJ, et al. Iatrogenic occlusion of the ophthalmic artery after cosmetic facial filler injections: a national survey by the Korean Retina Society. JAMA Ophthalmol 2014;132(6):714–23.

186. Coleman SR. Avoidance of arterial occlusion from injection of soft tissue fillers. Aesthet Surg J 2002;22(6):555–7.

187. Lee DH, Yang HN, Kim JC, et al. Sudden unilateral visual loss and brain infarction after autologous fat injection into nasolabial groove. Br J Ophthalmol 1996;80(11):1026.

188. Wu WT. The Oriental nose: an anatomical basis for surgery. Ann Acad Med Singap 1992;21(2):176–89.

189. Donofrio LM. Technique of periorbital lipoaugmentation. Dermatol Surg 2003;29(1):92–8.

190. DeLorenzi C. Complications of injectable fillers, part I. Aesthet Surg J 2013;33(4):561–75.

191. Douse-Dean T, Jacob CI. Fast and easy treatment for reduction of the Tyndall effect secondary to

cosmetic use of hyaluronic acid. J Drugs Dermatol 2008;7(3):281–3.

192. Fezza JP. Nonsurgical treatment of cicatricial ectropion with hyaluronic acid filler. Plast Reconstr Surg 2008;121(3):1009–14.

193. Hirsch RJ, Narurkar V, Carruthers J. Management of injected hyaluronic acid induced Tyndall effects. Lasers Surg Med 2006;38(3):202–4.

194. Braun M, Braun S. Nodule formation following lip augmentation using porcine collagen-derived filler. J Drugs Dermatol 2008;7(6):579–81.

195. Rossner M, Rossner F, Bachmann F, et al. Risk of severe adverse reactions to an injectable filler based on a fixed combination of hydroxyethylmethacrylate and ethylmethacrylate with hyaluronic acid. Dermatol Surg 2009;35: 367–74.

196. Wiest LG, Stolz W, Schroeder JA. Electron microscopic documentation of late changes in permanent fillers and clinical management of granulomas in affected patients. Dermatol Surg 2009;35:1681–8.

197. Narins RS. Minimizing adverse events associated with poly-L-lactic acid injection. Dermatol Surg 2008;34:S100–4.

198. Rossner F, Rossner M, Hartmann V, et al. Decrease of reported adverse events to injectable polylactic acid after recommending an increased dilution: 8-year results from the Injectable Filler Safety study. J Cosmet Dermatol 2009;8(1):14–8.

199. Sadick NS, Katz BE, Roy D. A multicenter, 47-month study of safety and efficacy of calcium hydroxylapatite for soft tissue augmentation of nasolabial folds and other areas of the face. Dermatol Surg 2007;33:S122–7.

200. Tzikas TL. Evaluation of the Radiance FN soft tissue filler for facial soft tissue augmentation. Arch Facial Plast Surg 2004;6(4):234–9.

201. Cohen JL. Understanding, avoiding, and managing dermal filler complications. Dermatol Surg 2008;34:S92–9.

202. Oranje AP, Folkers E, Choufoer-Habova J, et al. Diagnostic value of Tzanck smear in herpetic and non-herpetic vesicular and bullous skin disorders in pediatric practice. Acta Derm Venereol 1986; 66(2):127–33.

203. Niewiarowski S, Stuart RK, Thomas DP. Activation of intravascular coagulation by collagen. Proc Soc Exp Biol Med 1966;123(1):196–200.

204. Zillmann A, Luther T, Müller I, Kotzsch M, Spannagl M, Kauke T,, Engelmann B. Platelet-associated tissue factor contributes to the collagen-triggered activation of blood coagulation. Biochem Biophys Res Commun 2001;281(2): 603–9.

205. Engelmann B, Luther T, Müller I. Intravascular tissue factor pathway–a model for rapid initiation of coagulation within the blood vessel. Thromb Haemost 2003;89(01):3–8.

206. Leon C, Alex M, Klocke A, Morgenstern E, Moosbauer C, Eckly A,, Engelmann B. Platelet ADP receptors contribute to the initiation of intravascular coagulation. Blood 2004;103(2): 594–600.

207. Hofmann S, Huemer G, Kratochwill C, et al. Pathophysiology of fat embolisms in orthopedics and traumatology. Der Orthopade 1995;24(2):84–93.

208. Elmas E, Kälsch T, Suvajac N, et al. Activation of coagulation during alimentary lipemia under real-life conditions. Int J Cardiol 2007;114(2):172–5.

209. Shier MR, Wilson RF. Fat embolism syndrome: traumatic coagulopathy with respiratory distress. Surg Annu 1980;12:139–68.

210. Magnani A, Albanese A, Lamponi S, et al. Blood-interaction performance of differently sulphated hyaluronic acids. Thromb Res 1996;81(3):383–95.

211. Barbucci R, Lamponi S, Magnani A, et al. Influence of sulfation on platelet aggregation and activation with differentially sulfated hyaluronic acids. J Thromb Thrombolysis 1998;6(2):109–15.

212. Deutsch J. Severe local reaction to benzathine penicillin. A contribution to the Nicolau syndrome (dermatitis livedoides). Dtsch Gesundheitsw 1966;21(51):2433.

213. Lansky H. Nicolau syndrome from the viewpoint of the surgeon. Zentralblatt fur Chirurgie 1970;95(41): 1194–7.

214. Niedner A, Tiller R. Nicolau syndrome following retacillin compositum injection. Z arztliche Fortbildung 1970;64(1):39.

215. Schröter K, Lorenz K. Nicolau syndrome, form of drug-induced embolism.(Clinical picture–etiology and pathogenesis–prevention–comparison with Hoigné syndrome). Z arztliche Fortbildung 1971; 65(14):725–31.

216. Stiehl P, Weissbach G, Schröter K. Nicolau syndrome. Pathogenesis and clinical aspects of penicillin-induced arterial embolism. Schweizerische Medizinische Wochenschrift 1971;101(11):377.

217. Weinmann G, Schaefer L. Nicolau syndrome-a complication of depot-penicillin therapy. Acta Paediatr Acad Sci Hung 1977;18(1):41.

218. Meyer FU, Becker I. The origin and treatment of accidents after the injection of penicillin. Stomatologie der DDR 1978;28(2):119–23.

219. Taraszkiewicz F, Kiss B, Szorc W, et al. Nicolau syndrome. Polski tygodnik lekarski (Warsaw, Poland: 1960) 1979;34(45):1759–61.

220. Gebert K. Embolitic lumbar artery occlusion following benzathinpenicillin (penduran). A case contribution to Nicolau syndrome in adults.

Psychiatrie, Neurologie, medizinische Psychol 1980;32(7):443–6.

221. Modzelewska I, Dawidowicz-Szczepanowska A. Nicolau syndrome following administration of procaine penicillin. Wiad Lek 1980;33(3):231–3.

222. Stechły HJ. 2 cases of Nicolau syndrome in children. Pediatria polska 1982;57(4):267.

223. Anitua MS, de Pablos Guijarro JE, Ortega AN, et al. An extreme case of Nicolau syndrome. Angiologia 1983;35(2):73–85.

224. Müller-Vahl H. Aseptic tissue necrosis: a severe complication after intramuscular injections. Deutsche medizinische Wochenschrift (1946) 1984; 109(20):786–92.

Nasal Tip Deformities After Primary Rhinoplasty

Paul Bermudez, DMD, MD*, Faisal A. Quereshy, MD, DDS

KEYWORDS

- Rhinoplasty • Complications • Nasal tip • Bossae • Pinched • Ischemic • Overresected
- Pollybeak

KEY POINTS

- Because of the central location in the midface, even minimal nasal tip deformities may be noticed and upsetting to the patient.
- Prevention, early recognition, and, depending on the case, intervention are critical in minimizing these complications. If complications do occur, regular communication with the patient and follow-up are crucial.
- Secondary or revision rhinoplasties are not uncommon (5%–10%), and informing patients that future revision may be indicated should be a component of the informed consent process.
- Related to the nasal tip, deformities may include, but are not limited to, the presence of bossae, a pinched nasal tip, and an ischemic tip.

INTRODUCTION

Rhinoplasty is often considered the most challenging of all facial cosmetic procedures because of the central location of the nose in the midface making any deformity visible to the patient or viewer. In addition to being the most challenging, rhinoplasty is also one of the most popular facial cosmetic procedures, with an increasing number being performed annually. As the number of primary rhinoplasties performed continues to increase, one would expect that the number of patients seeking secondary or revision rhinoplasties would also increase. In the patient seeking secondary or revision rhinoplasty, deformities may be residual or iatrogenically induced. In a survey of surgeons, a self-reported revision rate of 0% to 5% was reported most commonly followed by a revision rate of 5% to 10%.[1] The reported revision rate finding reminds us that secondary or revision rhinoplasties are not uncommon, and informing patients that future revision may be indicated should be a component of the informed consent process. Related to the nasal tip, deformities may include, but are not limited to, the presence of bossae, a pinched nasal tip, and an ischemic tip. In addition, an overresected nose can affect multiple nasal structures, including the nasal tip. In a review by Nassab and Matti,[2] a large nasal tip was the chief complaint of 25% of patients presenting for evaluation for secondary or revision rhinoplasties. A large nasal tip was the second most common complaint after nasal asymmetry. A tip asymmetry was noted 26% of the time on clinical examination. A tip asymmetry was the third most common clinical finding after nostril asymmetry and septal deviation. Inadequate tip projection was present 20% of the time; an overprojected tip was present 14% of the time; and a pollybeak deformity was present 17% of the time. In addition to cosmetic deformities, a loss of function, such as difficulty with nasal breathing, was present in 22% of these patients. The diagnosis of nasal tip deformities will be discussed as well as remedies for treatment. Because of the proximity of the supratip

Department of Oral and Maxillofacial Surgery, Case Western Reserve University, 9601 Chester Avenue, Cleveland, OH 44106, USA
* Corresponding author.
E-mail address: pfb14@case.edu

Oral Maxillofacial Surg Clin N Am 33 (2021) 111–117
https://doi.org/10.1016/j.coms.2020.09.005
1042-3699/21/© 2020 Elsevier Inc. All rights reserved.

to the nasal tip, the supratip deformity (pollybeak deformity) will also be discussed.

ANATOMY

The terms nasal tip and nasal lobule are 2 terms used interchangeably to describe the most projected point of the nose. To avoid confusion, the term nasal tip will be used. Anatomically, the nasal tip is positioned between the 2 domes and between the supratip and infratip break. The nasal tip is often described as having 3 major tip supporters and 6 minor tip supporters. The major nasal tip supporters are the lower lateral cartilages, the attachment of the medial crura to the nasal septum, and the attachment of the lower and upper lateral cartilages. The minor tip supporters are the anterior nasal spine, the membranous nasal septum, the cartilaginous dorsal septum, the attachment of the soft tissue to the ala cartilages, the sesamoid cartilages, and the interdomal ligament between the lower lateral cartilages. The attachment of the lower and upper lateral cartilages, one of the major tip supporters, is termed the scroll area. The connection between the upper and lower lateral cartilages in the scroll has been described as interlocked, overlapping, end to end, or opposed. The lower lateral cartilages, one of the major tip supporters, are composed of the medial, intermediate, and lateral crus. The lower lateral cartilages also play an important role in supporting the external nasal valve. The left and right medial crus meet in the midline and attach to the nasal septum, making up the third major nasal tip support.[3]

PATIENT EVALUATION

In evaluating the patient considering a rhinoplasty, the patient's chief complaint should be carefully investigated as well as the patient's motivators for seeking treatment. Treatment in patients with external motivators should be avoided. Related to the nasal tip, common complaints include a bulbous or boxy nasal tip. Photograph documentation is crucial to assist in treatment planning. Photographs should be taken in the frontal view, profile view, and the worm's eye view. On clinical examination, the shape of the nasal tip should be evaluated. Nasal tip shapes include bulbous, pinched, twisted, asymmetric, and boxy. Nasal tip projection should also be evaluated. The Goode method is a commonly used method for evaluating nasal tip projection. In the Goode method, the nasal tip is measured from the alar point to the nasal tip (AP-NT). This is then divided by the distance from the nasion

to the nasal tip (N-NT). (AP-NT)/(N-NT) should ideally be between 0.55 and 0.60. The Crumley method is another method for evaluating nasal tip projection, and ideal proportions are based on a 3-4-5 triangle composed of AP-NT, N line (perpendicular to Frankfort horizontal)-AP, and N-NT. The presence of a supratip and infratip break as well as the tip defining point should be documented. From a worm's eye view, the ideal nasal base is triangular with alar margin support. The thickness of the skin overlying the nasal tip is important to evaluate. Changes in the underlying nasal tip anatomy are easily noticeable in patients with thin skin. Changes in the underlying nasal tip anatomy are less noticeable in patients with thick nasal skin.[3]

NASAL TIP DEFORMITIES
Bossae

Bossae are knoblike protuberances of the lower lateral cartilages that can occur after primary rhinoplasty (**Fig. 1**). Bossae is the plural of bossa, which is Latin for "bump." Bossae are best categorized as either early bossae or late bossae. Early bossae are those that occur within 3 months of primary rhinoplasty, and late bossae are those that occur greater than 1 year after primary rhinoplasty. Early bossae are often caused by either an uncorrected or an iatrogenically

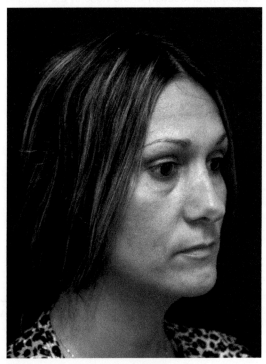

Fig. 1. Bossa over right nasal tip.

induced asymmetry. Late bossae, on the other hand, are caused by fibrosis or scar contracture on a weakened or unreconstituted cartilaginous framework. Patients with thin skin and strong cartilages are more prone to bossae formation. In order to prevent the formation of bossae, vestibular skin should be well undermined from strong asymmetric cartilages to prevent irregularities in the overlying skin. In patients with strong lower lateral cartilages, after septum exposure, the lower lateral cartilages should be well approximated with suturing techniques to prevent widening of the medial crura, which may lead to bossae formation. Overresection of the cephalic margins of the lower lateral cartilages should also be minimized, as this can lead to weakening of the lower lateral cartilages, buckling, and the formation of bossae. The recommendation is to leave at least 6 mm of the lower lateral cartilage intact to prevent buckling and bossae formation. Treatment of bossae includes further stabilization of the cartilages with suturing techniques or grafting. Shaving of the bossae should be avoided, as this further weakens the cartilage, one of the causative factors in bossae formation.[4]

Pinched Nasal Tip

A pinched nasal tip deformity is characterized by a clear demarcation between the nasal tip and the alar lobule, isolating the nasal tip from the rest of the nose. On frontal view, a pinched nasal tip can be seen as vertical shadows separating the nasal tip from the alar lobule. On worm's eye view, a pinched nasal tip is visualized as medial collapse of the alar margin and a loss of the normal triangular shape of the nasal base (**Fig. 2**). The pinched nasal tip is caused by tip modification techniques during primary rhinoplasty that attempt to narrow the nasal tip, resulting in weakened support to the alar margin causing medial collapse of

the alar lobule and tip pinching. The most common cause of a pinched nasal deformity is overresection of the cephalic edge of the lower lateral cartilages, resulting in weakening of the cartilage. At a minimum, 6 mm of cartilaginous support should be maintained.[5] In an ideal situation for alar margin support, the caudal margin of the lateral crus lies at the same level as the cephalic margin of the lateral crus. Common dome suturing methods used to narrow the nasal tip cinch the caudal margin of the lateral crus below the cephalic margin of the lateral crus, leading to a lack of alar margin support and an increased risk for a pinched nasal tip deformity.[6] Overprotrusive shield grafts may also lead to the appearance of a pinched nasal tip deformity. A pinched nasal tip may be minimized by properly contouring the graft at the time of placement. Separate from the cosmetic deformity caused by a pinched nasal tip, a functional complaint of decreased nasal breathing may occur due to the medial displacement of the alar lobule causing a decreased external nasal valve. The goals in treatment of the pinched nasal tip include restoring nasal tip contour and alar margin support. This is accomplished with the use of lateral crural strut grafts and alar rim grafts, which improve the strength of the alar margin and allows reestablishment of a more favorable relationship between the cephalic and caudal margins of the lateral crus. Less favorable effects that may be seen with lateral crural strut grafts include an increased nasal base width, flaring of the nostrils, and increased stiffness of the nose.[5,6]

Ischemic Tip

Nasal tip ischemia after primary rhinoplasty may occur due to overaggressive thinning of the nasal soft tissues, excessive tension on the skin after closure, and infection. It is important to recognize risk factors preoperatively that may increase the

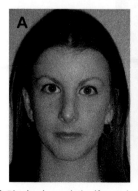
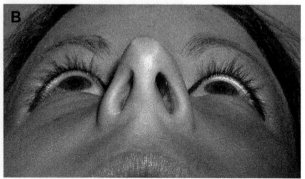

Fig. 2. (*A*) Pinched nasal tip (frontal view). (*B*) Pinched nasal tip (worm's eye view).

risk for nasal tip ischemia. These risks factors include smoking, previous rhinoplasty, history of head and neck radiation, use of vasconstrictive drugs, and systemic diseases that may contribute to peripheral vascular disease, including diabetes. Patients with a history of fillers may be at an increased risk for nasal tip ischemia. Related to the procedure itself, patients who undergo open rhinoplasty to increase the length of a short nose may be at an increased risk for nasal tip ischemia because of the increased tension on the skin after closure. Early recognition of nasal tip ischemia is important to prevent the loss of nasal tip skin (**Fig. 3**). Ischemia to the nasal tip can often become evident during closure of the transcolumellar incision during open rhinoplasty. If ischemia is evident during closure, the sutures should be removed and tension relieved. If ischemia is noted

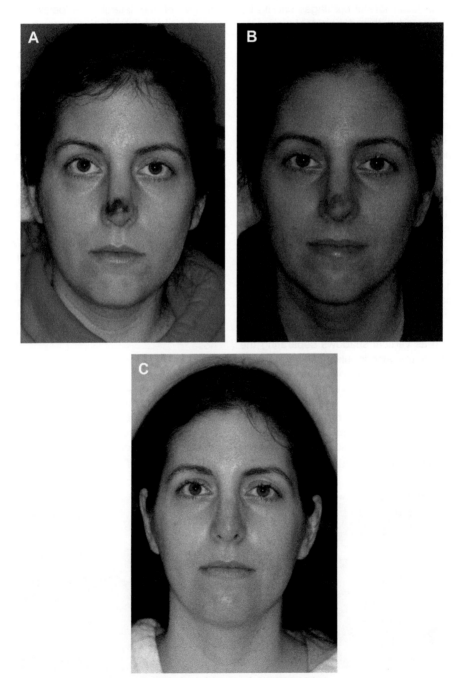

Fig. 3. (*A*) Initial ischemic tip. (*B*) Progress ischemic tip. (*C*) Resolving ischemic tip.

postoperatively or there remains a concern for nasal tip ischemia, 2% nitroglycerin ointment (Nitro-BID, Fougera Pharmaceutical Melville, NY, USA) can be applied topically twice daily for the next several days. In a recent case report, Amirlak and colleagues[7] used SPY Elite Laser Angiographic System (Stryker Corp, Novadaq Technologies, Kalamazoo, MI, USA) to analyze tissue perfusion after application of nitroglycerin paste during an open rhinoplasty. During the case, poor perfusion was noted clinically following placement of structural grafts at the nasal tip. Before removing the grafts, nitroglycerin paste was applied, and SPY was used to validate the effectiveness of the topical nitroglycerin on perfusion of the nasal tip. In this case, the grafts did not need to be removed. SPY uses properties of indocyanine green (ICG), a fluorescent agent with a half-life of 3 to 4 minutes. The contrast is administered intravenously and can be visualized in the deep dermis and subcutaneous vasculature. Because of the short half-life of ICG, the study can be repeated multiple times to evaluate changes in perfusion. If there is an increased concern for nasal tip ischemia, leech therapy can be used immediately postoperatively. Because of the presence of *Aeromonas hydrophila* within the leeches, antibiotic prophylaxis is necessary. Hyperbaric oxygen therapy can be an additional treatment modality, as well as daily aspirin, and the addition of pentoxifylline as a vasodilator. If necrosis of the nasal tip results, topical collagenase should be applied daily to debride the necrotic skin. Because nasal tip necrosis is an unacceptable complication of open rhinoplasty, prevention is critical. Patients scheduled for rhinoplasty should be urged to quit smoking 6 weeks before surgery. Intraoperatively, tension on the flap should be relieved periodically to prevent venous congestion. The use of electrocautery should be limited. Early recognition of ischemia should be identified during closure, and treatment should be initiated promptly. The use of Doyle splints should be avoided in patients with concern for nasal tip ischemia.[8]

Overresected Nose

In the past, primary rhinoplasty techniques often included a largely resective technique in an attempt to make a more defined nose. These overaggressive techniques often resulted in an overresected nose. A largely resective technique has fallen out of favor, and a more conservative technique with focus on preserving the nasal structures is used today. Although resective techniques are less commonly used, the surgeon performing secondary rhinoplasties will likely treat patients with a history of a primary rhinoplasty that resulted in an overresected nose. In a retrospective review, Nassab and Matti[2] noted that 26% of patients presenting for secondary rhinoplasties had an overresected nose. Although the overresected nose is not specific to the nasal tip, an overresected nose unquestionably affects the nasal tip. The overresected components of the nose may include the nasal septum, the nasal dorsum, the upper and lower nasal cartilages, and the alar rim. In regard to the nasal tip, an overresected nasal septum may result in loss of nasal tip projection; an overresected dorsum may result in an excessive supratip break or supratip deformity, and an overresected lower lateral cartilage may result in a pinched nasal tip. An overresected nasal septum can be treated with a septal extension graft.[9] An overresected dorsum can be treated with dorsal augmentation using various techniques. In a 2019 review, Nassimizadeh and colleagues[10] recommended the use of diced autogenous cartilage wrapped in temporalis fascia, which can be placed along the nasal dorsum. A pinched nasal tip can be treated with a combination of columella strut grafting, nasal tip grafts, and suturing techniques, as discussed earlier.

Supratip Deformity (Pollybeak Deformity)

A common complication of primary rhinoplasty is a supratip deformity, which is identified by fullness in the supratip region. Because this may resemble a parrot's beak, it has also been known as a pollybeak deformity (**Fig. 4**).[11] Although the supratip deformity is most commonly identified as a complication of primary rhinoplasty, it may also be present before treatment. In patients presenting for evaluation for rhinoplasty, Guyuron and colleagues[12] noted a pollybeak deformity in 9% of primary rhinoplasty candidates and in 36% of secondary rhinoplasty candidates. In patients with secondary deformities, the supratip deformity was caused by an overresected caudal dorsum (30%), an underresected caudal dorsum (30%), an underprojected tip (15%), or a combination of these factors. In patients undergoing secondary rhinoplasty, a significant amount of fibrosis was noted in the supratip region compared with those patients undergoing primary rhinoplasty. The excess fibrosis was attributed to the failure to reduce dead space during the primary rhinoplasty. To avoid the development of a supratip deformity, proper reduction of the caudal dorsum was recommended, avoidance of dead space and the development or

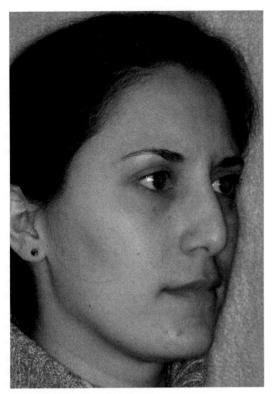

Fig. 4. Pollybeak deformity.

preservation of adequate nasal tip projection. A supratip suture approximating the supratip subcutaneous tissue to the underlying cartilage was used. A protocol for management of the supratip deformity was recommended. If the development of collapsible supratip tissue was noted postoperatively, aggressive taping to reduce dead space was recommended for a period of 4 weeks. If taping did not improve the deformity, then the injection of a low volume of triamcinolone 4 to 8 mg was recommended in the deep tissues monthly for up to 3 months. If triamcinolone injections did not improve the deformity, then the final option was a revision rhinoplasty in 1 year. For patients requiring revision rhinoplasty, resection of excess soft tissue, placement of supratip cartilage graft to remove dead space, and supratip suture were advised. If the deformity was due to underresection of the caudal dorsum, then additional resection was recommended. If the deformity was due to an underprojected nasal tip, then additional tip augmentation was advised.[12] It is important to note that an individual patient's tissues may react differently to surgery, and the postoperative results may be difficult to predict. Patient variability is seen in the work of Hussein and colleagues,[13] whereby an increased risk for a supratip deformity (62%) was seen in Middle

Eastern patients presenting for secondary rhinoplasty. The increased risk for a supratip deformity was attributed to an increased thickness of the skin and increased number of sebaceous glands in the Middle Eastern population, which may be attributed to increased postoperative edema and fibrosis. Hussein and colleagues, findings differ from that of Nassab and Matti,[2] who in the United Kingdom noted a supratip deformity in 17% of the patients presenting for evaluation for secondary rhinoplasty.

SUMMARY

Nasal tip deformities after primary rhinoplasty may occur, including the formation of bossae, a pinched nasal tip, and nasal tip ischemia. In addition, an overresected nose may affect the nasal tip, and a lack of tip support may contribute to a supratip deformity. Because of the central location in the midface, even minimal nasal tip deformities (small bossa) may be noticed and upsetting to the patient. In addition to minimal nasal tip deformities, more severe nasal tip deformities, including nasal tip ischemia, are easily visible to any viewer. Prevention, early recognition, and, depending on the case, intervention are critical in minimizing these complications. If complications do occur, regular communication with the patient and follow-up are crucial.

CLINICS CARE POINTS

- The thickness of the skin overlying the nasal tip is important to evaluate. Changes in the underlying nasal tip anatomy are easily noticeable in patients with thin skin. Changes in the underlying nasal tip anatomy are less noticeable in patients with thick skin.
- Patients with thin skin and strong cartilages are more prone to bossae formation. In order to prevent the formation of bossae, vestibular skin should be well undermined from strong asymmetric cartilages to prevent irregularities in the overlying skin.
- Overresection of the cephalic margins should be minimized as this can lead to weakening of the lower lateral cartilages. The recommendation is to leave at least 6 mm of the lower lateral cartilage intact to prevent buckling.
- Nasal tip ischemia can often become evident during closure of the transcolumellar incision during open rhinoplasty. If ischemia is evident during closure, the sutures should be removed and tension relieved.

- Due to the risk for ischemia, patients scheduled for rhinoplasty should be urged to quit smoking 6 weeks before surgery.

DISCLOSURE

The authors have nothing to disclose.

REFERENCES

1. Warner J, Gutowski K, Shama L, et al. National Interdisciplinary Rhinoplasty Survey. Aesthet Surg J 2009;29(94):295–301.
2. Nassab R, Matti M. Presenting concerns and surgical management of secondary rhinoplasty. Aesthet Surg J 2015;35(2):137–44.
3. Cuzalinia A. Ch. 8 rhinoplasty cosmetic facial surgery. New York: Elsevier; 2011. p. 175–246.
4. Kridel RWH, Yoon PJ, Koch RJ. Prevention and correction of nasal tip bossae in rhinoplasty. Arch Facial Plast Surg 2003;5:416–22.
5. Paun SH, Trenite GN. Correction of the pinched nasal tip deformity. Ch 19 Master techniques in rhinoplasty. Philadelphia: Elsevier Health Sciences; 2011.
6. Ari H, Khayat ST. Correction of nasal pinching. Facial Plast Surg Clin North Am 2019;27:477–89.
7. Amirlak B, Dehdashitian A, Sanneic K, et al. Unique uses of spy: revision rhinoplasty. Plast Reconstr Surg Glob Open 2019;7(6):e2123.
8. Kerolous JL, Nassif PS. Treatment protocol for compromised nasal skin. Facial Plast Surg Clin North Am 2019;27:505–11.
9. Hubbard T. Exploiting the septum for maximum control. Ann Plast Surg 2000;44:173–80.
10. Nassimizadeh A, Nassimizadeh M, Wu J, et al. Correction of the overresected nose. Facial Plast Surg Clin North Am 2019;27:451–63.
11. Rohrich RJ, Shanmugakrishnan RR, Mohan R. Rhinoplasty refinements: addressing the pollybeak deformity. Plast Reconstr Surg 2020;145(3):696–9.
12. Guyuron B, DeLuca L, Lash R. Supratip deformity: a closer look. Plast Reconstr Surg 2000;105(3):1140–51.
13. Hussein W, Foda H. Pollybeak deformity in middle eastern rhinoplasty: prevention and treatment. Facial Plast Surg 2016;32(4):398–401.

Correction of Septal Perforation/Nasal Airway Repair

Keith A. Sonneveld, DDS[a],*, Pradeep K. Sinha, MD, PhD[b]

KEYWORDS

- Septal perforation • Internal nasal valve • External nasal valve • Septoplasty • Nasal airway

KEY POINTS

- Rhinoplasty is a procedure that has potential to compromise or potentially enhance the nasal airway.
- Diagnosis of preoperative nasal airway compromise can help inform treatment to preclude complications involving the nasal airway.
- Intimate knowledge of airway manipulation and grafting techniques can elevate the rhinoplasty surgeon and their patient care.
- Septal surgery poses a risk of septal perforation if the mucoperichondrium does not remain intact.
- Many techniques have been described to repair septal perforation; however, no techniques have shown superiority over another.

INTRODUCTION

Rhinoplasty is typically thought of as a cosmetic procedure; however, treatment can have significantly implications for the function of the nasal airway. Nasal obstruction is a common complaint. An esthetically pleasing outcome that significantly compromises nasal airway function may be considered as an unsuccessful result by some surgeons. A recent survey of plastic surgeons shows that nearly 40% of surgeons report difficulty breathing post-rhinoplasty in more than 20% of patients and that almost 30% of these surgeons do not consider themselves to be adequately trained in assessing and managing the airway during a rhinoplasty.[1] The surgeon performing a rhinoplasty procedure must be cognizant of the nasal airway and the effects that their manipulations and alterations in the structure can have on the nasal airway.

CAUSES OF NASAL AIRWAY COMPROMISE

Classically the most commonly recognized causes of anatomically based nasal airway obstruction (NAO) have been recognized as related to abnormalities in one or more of the following structures[2]:

- External nasal valve (ENV)
- Internal nasal valve (INV)
- Nasal septum
- Inferior turbinate

There are multiple causes of NAO other than anatomic abnormalities[s]; however, discussion of these other causes is not included in the scope of this work. The work by Villwock and Kuppersmith[3] is a good reference for these other considerations and offers an algorithm for differentiation between causes of NAO.

The ENV is the most caudal aspect of the external nares, and the structures that compromise the ENV include the lateral crus of the lower

[a] FACES Fort Worth, 4421 Oak Park Ln Ste 101, Fort Worth, TX 76109, USA; [b] Atlanta Institute for Facial Aesthetic Surgery, 5730 Glenridge Drive, Suite T200, Atlanta, GA 30328, USA
* Corresponding author.
E-mail address: KSonneveld@live.com

Oral Maxillofacial Surg Clin N Am 33 (2021) 119–124
https://doi.org/10.1016/j.coms.2020.09.006

lateral cartilage (LLC), the medial crus of the LLC, the nasal septum, and the floor of the nose.[4] ENV collapse is caused by an inherent lack of structural integrity, overresection during rhinoplasty, and destabilization during rhinoplasty.

The INV is the middle third of the nasal vault and is made up of the upper lateral cartilage (ULC), the nasal septum, the nasal floor, and the inferior turbinate (**Fig. 1**).[2] INV collapse is characterized by a decrease in the angle formed between the septum and the ULC, which is typically 10° to 15°.[5]

The nasal septum is a composite structure made of the quadrangular cartilage, the perpendicular plate of the ethmoid bone, and the vomer bone (**Fig. 2**). Deviation in the nasal septum away from midline can compromise airflow through the nasal airway. Nasal septal deviation is acquired or congenital in nature.

The inferior turbinate is a component of the latera nasal wall, which can hypertrophy and cause a nasal obstruction. The nature of the turbinate hypertrophy may be bony, submucosal, or a combination of both. Often the inferior turbinate hypertrophies in areas opposite the side of nasal septal deviation.

A combination of the ENV and the INV has been referred to as the nasal inlet.[6] This composite structure has influences on the nasal airflow based on the size of the aperture. Although the following discussion is an oversimplification of the airflow within the nasal airway, it can help to conceptualize the ideal approach to the nasal airway during rhinoplasty. Poiseuille equation $\left(R = \frac{8nL}{\pi r^4}\right)$ regarding flow dynamics shows that flow and pressure is related to airway resistance, length, and radius (Darcy–Weisbach equation can be further applied). Because of the exponential component of the radius variable, changes in this variable have an amplified effect on resistance to flow.

By the same token, Bernoulli principle relates that flow differential between different areas can create a negative pressure effect.[7] The negative pressure can create a collapse of the ENV and/or the INV, creating a decrease in the radius of the nasal inlet. Structural strength helps resist collapse in response to negative airway pressure.[8]

Historically reductive rhinoplasty is associated with decrease in ENV and long-term dissatisfaction with nasal airflow. This is often related to overresection of the LLC for tip refinement, causing weakening of the cartilage or alar scarring and retraction, thereby narrowing the ENV.[9–11] Destabilization of the cartilaginous components without proper resuspension or reinforcement has been implicated in postoperative NAO.[11]

A retrospective review of several-hundred patients who have had nasal airway repair surgery showed that long-term postoperative moderate or severe NAO was reported at 82%. It also discussed that nasal valve collapse was present but not treated in patients who had septoplasty/turbinoplasty with no satisfactory improvement in airway obstruction.[12] Nasal valve compromise has been reported to be responsible for 70% of nasal resistance.[13]

NAO can exist in a patient who has had rhinoplasty or someone who has not had rhinoplasty before. Proper diagnosis dictates the proper treatment plan for these patients. A patient-tailored approach to treatment of source of NAO yielded improved results.[14]

Patient history and physical examination are important in determining the cause of NAO. Examination can include several methods including palpation to evaluate the structural integrity of cartilage and the cartilaginous junctions, anterior rhinoscopy using a nasal speculum, nasal endoscopy when indicated, acoustic rhinometry, and

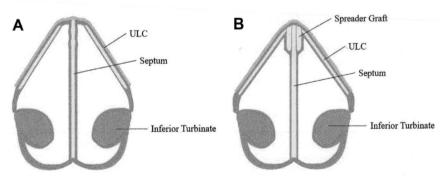

Fig. 1. (*A*) Diagrammatic representation of the internal nasal valve, demonstrating an approximate relationship between the ULC, the nasal septum, the inferior turbinate, and the nasal floor. (*B*) Spreader grafts are placed on each side of the nasal septum to increase the angle between the ULC and the nasal septum.

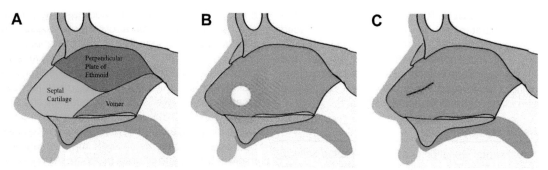

A

Perpendicular
Plate of
Ethmoid

Septal
Cartilage

Vomer

B

C

Fig. 2. (*A*) The nasal septum has bony and cartilaginous components as noted in this diagram. (*B*) This diagram shows an anteriorly located perforation. Incision is made circumferentially around the perforation and subperiochondrial undermining is carried out as noted with the *red hash marks* and is advanced for primary closure. (*C*) The local advancement flap is sutured with a fast resorbable suture. If the contralateral nasal mucosa is advanced for closure (with or without interposing tissue graft), then it is imperative to create incision closure lines that do not oppose each other.

the Cottle maneuver to evaluate nasal valve function. These all help to determine diagnosis; however, no consensus exists as to which test is best for evaluating nasal valve function.[7]

TREATMENT OF NASAL AIRWAY OBSTRUCTION

Although a focus of this article is discussion of the complications relating to rhinoplasty, it is recognized that secondary repair of a nasal airway following rhinoplasty is similar to the repair of a nasal airway without a history of previous rhinoplasty. Nasal valve compromise, whether it is the ENV or INV, following rhinoplasty is often related to overresection of cartilage, destabilization without proper resuspension of structures, and failure to recognize an inherent lack of structural integrity.

Different options exist for treatment of nasal valve collapse including spreader graft, batten grafts, alar valve suspension, and splay grafts.[10,13] Evidence is lacking to demonstrate superiority of one method of INV repair compared with other methods; however, currently spreader grafts are considered the gold standard for nasal valve repair.[15] The following discussion of treatment options is colored with the perspective of the senior author (P.K.S.) and treatment of NAO.

A complicating factor in treating post-rhinoplasty nasal obstruction is the difficulty obtaining graft material. If the patient has had previous rhinoplasty and/or septoplasty, it is likely that the septal cartilage has been manipulated in some way. This has implications in the quantity and quality of the cartilage available for harvest. If the septal cartilage is insufficient for reconstructive grafting, then other sites for cartilage harvest must be considered, including auricular cartilage

and rib cartilage.[16] Composite grafts may be useful in alar retraction. Alloplastic grafts and xenografts may also be considered but are generally less preferable than autogenous grafts.

External Nasal Valve

Treatment of ENV collapse often includes reconstructing the LLC to a state of increased strength and/or resuspension to an appropriate level. Alar batten grafts are used to increase the length and strengthen the latera crus of the LLC and are placed as an overlay or underlay.[17] An underlay graft is more esthetically pleasing, but an overlay graft typically imparts more structural integrity. The graft can extend to the lateral nasal wall, where it is secured to the periosteum of the piriform rim or it is placed into a soft tissue pocket laterally.

If the source of the collapse is not related to the strength of the cartilage itself, but rather disarticulation between the ULC and the LLC, the cartilage may be resuspended following dissection of the cartilage from the mucoperiosteum.

Internal Nasal Valve

Dorsal hump reduction during rhinoplasty can compromise the attachment of the ULC to the nasal septum, which can cause an inferior and medial displacement of the ULC. This can cause a decrease in the nasal valve angle, thereby compromising airflow through the nasal airway.

The most common method of INV collapse is placement of spreader grafts. Spreader grafts are used to create dorsal aesthetic units, to support a longer nose length, and to increase the nasal tip projection in secondary and tertiary rhinoplasty cases.[16] The spreader graft is fashioned ideally 3 to 4 mm in height and spans the same length as the ULC. The ULC and nasal septum is then separated, and the graft cartilage is placed immediately lateral to the nasal septal cartilage bilaterally in a submucoperichondrial pocket, and the graft cartilage is secured to the septal cartilage using a slow resorbing or permanent suture in a horizontal mattress fashion (see **Fig. 1**).

Nasal Septum

Nasal septal deviation is a common issue seen in practice. This is primarily present, post-traumatic and post-rhinoplasty. The septum is a composite structure composed of bony and cartilaginous structures, which are ideally both addressed in a septoplasty. The nasal septum is often used as the site for cartilage harvest for grafting in the rhinoplasty. Cartilaginous septum is displaced off the maxillary crest, and it can also have significant deviation caused by buckling or defects in the structural integrity of the cartilage itself.

The septum is primarily addressed at our institution through a Killian incision, and subperichondrial dissection is carried out through the extent of the cartilaginous septum and continued subperiosteally to expose the bony septum. The quadrangular cartilage is then disarticulated from the bony septum. Becker double-action septum scissors are used to create a controlled cut at the superior aspect of a deviation to prevent aberrant fractures that involve the cribriform plate. The deviated portion of the bony septum is then addressed by removal with a double-action punch or Takahashi forceps. Four-millimeter osteotomes are used to remove bony spurs that may exist on the nasal floor.

The cartilaginous septum is then addressed. In cases of primary rhinoplasty the posterior-inferior septum is harvested and saved for grafting during rhinoplasty. Typically, the septum is harvested in a fashion that preserves an L-strut of the dorsal and caudal septum with a dimension of no less than 20 mm, but typically greater. In isolated septoplasty, cartilage may be harvested and/or morselized to remove the deviations. It is usually replaced into the subperiosteal pocket before incision closure. If there is a dislocation of the cartilaginous septum in the anterior aspect, it is secured to the maxillary crest using a long-term resorbable suture to the periosteum.

Inferior Turbinate

Addressing hypertrophy is done by several methods. Total (not preferable) and partial turbinectomy has been described, although the development of atrophic rhinitis, also known as ozena or "empty-nose syndrome," is a potential complication. Turbinectomy addresses soft tissue and hard tissue concerns, but other methods are used to address the individual components.

Several modalities are used to perform submucous resection of the hypertrophied soft tissue including manual instrumentation, microdebrider, electrocautery, laser, and radiofrequency ablation. Meta-analysis of the literature showed outcomes comparing these different modalities. The greatest percentage of patients showed improvement with microdebrider, and poorest percentage of patients showed improvement with manual instrumentation and cryotherapy.[18]

The bony component when not treated as a turbinectomy is performed with turbinate outfracture, which is achieved with a broad instrument out-fracturing the bone to a more lateral position against the nasal wall. Bony reduction can also be achieved with submucous resection.[18,19]

NASAL SEPTAL PERFORATION

Nasal septal perforation is a condition that can present with pain, bleeding, nasal obstruction, crusting, and whistling sounds from the nose. The prevalence of nasal septal perforation has been reported to be 0.9% in the general population. A study of computed tomography scans in an urban population showed the prevalence to be 2.05%, and of these patients, 3 of 76 were noted to have a history of facial surgery.[20] In a review of a 31-year history of septal perforation repair, 62.4% of patients presented with a history of previous rhinoplasty and/or septoplasty.[21] A recent meta-analysis of nasal surgery complications reports an incidence of septal perforation from 0% to 2.6%.[22]

The vascular supply to the mucoperichondrium is from branches of the internal and external carotid arteries and can cause ischemia to the tissue when vascular compromise occurs, in cases of vasculitis and trauma. With ischemia and/or exposure of the underlying septal quandrangular cartilage, necrosis of the cartilage occurs.[23]

The normal laminar airflow that occurs in a nose is thus disrupted, which can create dryness and irritation that can result in crusting around the perforation. Chronic irritation and manipulation of this crust may increase the size of the perforation.[23,24] Other complications from a septal perforation may range from minor irritation and perichondritis to chronic epistaxis and loss of septal support, which can result in loss of nasal tip support and a saddle nose deformity.[23,25] Septal perforation may go unnoticed in patients up to 39% of the time.[26]

Evaluation includes a history of past surgeries including rhinoplasty and septoplasty. There are multiple causes of septal perforation, which include postsurgical, traumatic,[27] inflammatory (sarcoidosis, Churg-Strauss syndrome, polyangiitis granulomatosis, lupus), infectious (septal abscess, tuberculosis, syphilis), malignancy, and inhaled substances.[23,24] A nasal endoscopy is recommended for evaluation of the anatomy of the nasal cavity and to measure the size of the defect, because this may change treatment planning for repair of defect if indicated. It is imperative to evaluate for other potential causes of septal defect.

Nonsurgical Management

Initial steps in nonsurgical management include patient counseling to minimize further iatrogenic trauma from digital or exogenous manipulation of the defect. Hygiene of the area should proceed primarily with saline irrigation of the area. Using a lubricant or ointment may prevent from drying the tissue if applied several times daily. If the tissue shows active inflammation as noted on nasal endoscopy an antibacterial ointment may be advisable.

Nasal septal button may also be used as a nonsurgical method for management of a septal perforation and is easily placed in clinic under local or topical anesthetic.[28,29] The device is placed with flanges on either side and may be left for up to a year, although some indications for removal of the device include an inability to provide proper hygiene, persistent pain, and increasing size of the defect.

Surgical Management

The current state of the literature does not show any consensus recommendations on surgical management for perforations. However, a systematic review showed that the success of repair in perforations less than 2 cm was 93% and decreased to 78% in perforations greater than 2 cm, but this did not control for the different techniques used.[30]

Most techniques described stress obtaining primary closure, whether it is unilateral or bilateral primary closure (see **Fig. 2**). Multiple different flap techniques, random pattern and axial flaps, have been described.[31–37] A controversial aspect of the closure technique is the use of an intervening graft material between flaps to make a 3-layer closure. Also described are use of acellular dermis solely to reconstruct the defect, which is only recommended in small perforations.[38] Temporalis fascia, cartilage, and polydioxanone plates have been reported for use in between opposing primary closure

using local flaps.[39–41] A systematic review suggests that interpositional grafts reduce failure rate of perforation repair; however, the controversy remains regarding its usefulness.[30]

In cases where previous septoplasty or rhinoplasty was performed, often the septum is harvested for grafting purposes and is scarce beneath the mucoperichondrium or even absent adjacent to the perforation.[24] This makes dissection of the flaps much more difficult.

Nasal septal perforations are an unfortunate but rare complication of nasal surgery, which has an overall good prognosis with proper patient counseling and cessation of habits that can only exacerbate the condition. Knowledge of the nonsurgical and surgical management can enhance patient care by execution of the proper treatment plan or by referral to a surgeon capable of management.

CLINICS CARE POINTS

- Overlooking the functional status of the nose can be a major pitfall when considering cosmetic nasal surgery.
- Early treatment of functional nasal deficits can often be more easily treated than secondary reconstruction of deficits following cosmetic surgery.
- Mobilization of vascular tissue to obturate a nasal septal perforation is absolutely imperative to achieve successful closure of an NSP.

DISCLOSURE

The authors have nothing to disclose.

REFERENCES

1. Afifi AM, Kempton SJ, Gordon CR, et al. Evaluating current functional airway surgery during rhinoplasty: a survey of the American Society of Plastic Surgeons. Aesthetic Plast Surg 2015;39(2):181–90.
2. Hsu DW, Suh JD. Anatomy and physiology of nasal obstruction. Otolaryngol Clin North Am 2018;51(5):853–65.
3. Villwock JA, Kuppersmith RB. Diagnostic algorithm for evaluating nasal airway obstruction. Otolaryngol Clin North Am 2018;51(5):867–72.
4. Ishii LE, Tollefson TT, Basura GJ, et al. Clinical practice guideline: improving nasal form and function after rhinoplasty executive summary. Otolaryngol Head Neck Surg 2017;156(2):205–19.
5. Ghosh A, Friedman O. Surgical treatment of nasal obstruction in rhinoplasty. Clin Plast Surg 2019;43(1):29–40.
6. Naughton JP, Lee AY, Ramos E, et al. Effect of nasal valve shape on downstream volume, airflow, and

pressure drop: importance of the nasal valve revisited. Ann Otol Rhinol Laryngol 2018;127(11):745–53.

7. Ishii LE, Rhee JS. Are diagnostic tests useful for nasal valve compromise? Laryngoscope 2013;123(1):7–8.

8. Zoumalan RA, Larrabee WF, Murakami CS. Intraoperative suction-assisted evaluation of the nasal valve in rhinoplasty. Arch Facial Plast Surg 2012;14(1):34–8.

9. Timperley D, Stow N, Srubiski A, et al. Functional outcomes of structured nasal tip refinement. Arch Facial Plast Surg 2010;12(5):298–304.

10. Friedman O, Cekic E, Gunel C. Functional rhinoplasty. Facial Plast Surg Clin North Am 2017;25(2):195–9.

11. Nadimi S, Kim DW. Revision functional surgery: salvaging function. Facial Plast Surg Clin North Am 2017;25(2):251–62.

12. Clark DW, Del Signore AG, Raithatha R, et al. Nasal airway obstruction: prevalence and anatomic contributors. Ear. Nose Throat J 2018;97(6):173–6.

13. Kenyon GS, Andrew P. Nasal valve surgery. Rhinol Facial Plast Surg 2009;75–81. https://doi.org/10.1007/978-3-540-74380-4_5.

14. Akduman D, Yanilmaz M, Haksever M, et al. Patients' evaluation for the surgical management of nasal obstruction. Rhinology 2013;51(4):361–7.

15. Goudakos JK, Fishman JM, Patel K. A systematic review of the surgical techniques for the treatment of internal nasal valve collapse: where do we stand? Clin Otolaryngol 2017;42(1):60–70.

16. Ors S. Osseous-cartilaginous spreader graft and nasal framework reconstruction. Aesthetic Plast Surg 2017;41(5):1155–63.

17. Chua DY, Park SS. Alar batten grafts. JAMA Facial Plast Surg 2014;16(5):377–8.

18. Sinno S, Mehta K, Lee ZH, et al. Inferior turbinate hypertrophy in rhinoplasty: systematic review of surgical techniques. Plast Reconstr Surg 2016;138(3):419e–29e.

19. Downs BW. The inferior turbinate in rhinoplasty. Facial Plast Surg Clin North Am 2017;25(2):171–7.

20. Gold M, Boyack I, Caputo N, et al. Imaging prevalence of nasal septal perforation in an urban population. Clin Imaging 2017;43(2017):80–2.

21. Kridel RWH, Delaney SW. Simultaneous septal perforation repair with septorhinoplasty: a 31-year experience. Facial Plast Surg 2018;1(212):298–311.

22. Sharif-Askary B, Carlson AR, Van Noord MG, et al. Incidence of post-operative adverse events after rhinoplasty. Plast Reconstr Surg 2019;(1):1.

23. Watson D, Barkdull G. Surgical management of the septal perforation. Otolaryngol Clin North Am 2009;42(3):483–93.

24. Kridel RWH, Delaney SW. Approach to correction of septal perforation. Facial Plast Surg Clin North Am 2019;27(4):443–9.

25. Robitschek J, Hilger P. The saddle deformity: camouflage and reconstruction. Facial Plast Surg Clin North Am 2017;25(2):239–50.

26. Lanier B, Kai G, Marple B, et al. Pathophysiology and progression of nasal septal perforation. Ann Allergy Asthma Immunol 2007;99(6):473–80.

27. Bakshi SS, Coumare VN, Priya M, et al. Long-term complications of button batteries in the nose. J Emerg Med 2016;50(3):485–7.

28. Abbas J, Anari S. Septal button insertion: the two-forcep screw technique. Laryngoscope 2013;123(5):1119–20.

29. Taylor RJ, Sherris DA. Prosthetics for nasoseptal perforations: a systematic review and meta-analysis. Otolaryngol Head Neck Surg 2015;152(5):803–10.

30. Kim SW, Rhee CS. Nasal septal perforation repair: predictive factors and systematic review of the literature. Curr Opin Otolaryngol Head Neck Surg 2012;20(1):58–65.

31. Re M, Paolucci L, Romeo R, et al. Surgical treatment of nasal septal perforations. Our experience. Acta Otorhinolaryngol Ital 2006;26(2):102–9.

32. Virkkula P, Mäkitie A Makatite, Vento SI. Surgical outcome and complications of nasal septal perforation repair with temporal fascia and periosteal grafts. Clin Med Insights Ear Nose Throat 2015;8. CMENT.S23230.

33. Islam A, Celik H, Felek SA, et al. Repair of nasal septal perforation with "cross-stealing" technique. Am J Rhinol Allergy 2009;23(2):225–8.

34. Cavada MN, Orgain CA, Alvarado R, et al. Septal perforation repair utilizing an anterior ethmoidal artery flap and collagen matrix. Am J Rhinol Allergy 2019;33(3):256–62.

35. Chen FH, Rui X, Deng J, et al. Endoscopic sandwich technique for moderate nasal septal perforations. Laryngoscope 2012;122(11):2367–72.

36. Presutti L, Ciufelli MA, Marchioni D, et al. Nasal septal perforations: our surgical technique. Otolaryngol Head Neck Surg 2007;136(3):369–72.

37. Tasca I, Compadretti GC. Closure of nasal septal perforation via endonasal approach. Otolaryngol Head Neck Surg 2006;135(6):922–7.

38. Sharma A, Janus J, Diggelmann HR, et al. Healing septal perforations by secondary intention using acellular dermis as a bioscaffold. Ann Otol Rhinol Laryngol 2015;124(6):425–9.

39. Sand JP, Desai SC, Branham GH. Septal perforation repair using polydioxanone plates: a 10-year comparative study. Plast Reconstr Surg 2015;136(4):700–3.

40. Cassano M. Riparazione della perforazione del setto nasale con tecnica endoscopica. Acta Otorhinolaryngol Ital 2017;37(6):486–92.

41. Conrad DJ, Zhang H, Côté DWJ. Acellular human dermal allograft as a graft for nasal septal perforation reconstruction. Plast Reconstr Surg 2018;141(6):1517–24.

Correction of the Overly Shortened Nose

Grace Lee Peng, MD[a],*, Babak Azizzadeh, MD[b]

KEYWORDS

- Overly shortened nose • Foreshortened nose • Overrotated nasal tip • Rib cartilage graft
- Cartilage grafting for revision rhinoplasty • Caudal septal extension graft • Cartilage grafting
- Nasal reconstruction

KEY POINTS

- The overly shortened nose is often caused by previous surgery.
- Causes for an overly shortened nose include contraction of the skin as well as scarring after initial or previous rhinoplasties.
- Correction of the overly shortened nose often includes costal cartilage grafting.
- Preoperative discussion of goals for the surgery allows for management of patients' expectations.

INTRODUCTION

The overly shortened nose can often be a complication from prior rhinoplasty surgery or from congenital and traumatic causes. Nasal length is usually described as the distance from the glabella to the subnasale, and its ideal length is when it is one-third the length of a person's face.[1] An overly shortened nose is often paired with an upturned and overrotated nasal tip. For men, the ideal aesthetic for the nasolabial angle should be anywhere from 90 to 105°, whereas for women, it is 95 to 115°.[2]

In this article, we discuss the correction of the short nose deformity after previous rhinoplasty and the techniques used by both authors. Historically, rhinoplasties were often reductive in nature to achieve the desired aesthetic goals. We have since found that reductive rhinoplasties can lead to many issues of nasal valve collapse as well as issues of tip deviation, overrotation, and overshortening of the nose.[3]

PREOPERATIVE ANALYSIS

The preoperative evaluation is critically important. Standardized preoperative photographs are taken the clinic during both the consultation as well as the preoperative appointment. At the time of the consultation, the patient is examined in the clinic room and the septum is palpated as well as the nose and nasal skin and soft tissue envelope. This is to evaluate the amount of remaining septal cartilage from previous rhinoplasty as well as gauge the ability of the skin to stretch as the nose is lengthened in surgery.

One of the major limitations during the correction of the overly shortened nose is the quality of the skin and its ability to cover over the area of grafting once the nose is lengthened and be able to close at the transcolumellar incision without tension. The limitations can be the scar tissue of the skin, lack of skin due to previous resection, or very thick skin that is already tight over the nasal dorsum and tip. Skin that is excessively scarred down to the underlying framework needs to also

[a] Facial Plastic and Reconstructive Surgery, 120 South Spalding Drive, Suite 301, Beverly Hills, CA 90212, USA;
[b] Center for Advanced Facial Plastic Surgery, 9401 Wilshire Boulevard, Suite 650, Beverly Hills, CA 90212, USA
* Corresponding author.
E-mail address: drpeng@graceleepengmd.com

Oral Maxillofacial Surg Clin N Am 33 (2021) 125–129
https://doi.org/10.1016/j.coms.2020.09.011
1042-3699/21/© 2020 Elsevier Inc. All rights reserved.

be noted, as that skin will have a higher chance for issues with vascularity and perfusion postoperatively.

Should skin appear to be too tight to be able to allow for adequate lengthening, the patient can help to stretch out the skin by pulling down caudally and exercising the skin to loosen it. It is also important to evaluate other procedures that will be done simultaneously that will help to provide some skin laxity, which can include deprojection of the tip or decreasing the height of the dorsal profile. Surgery should be performed only once the skin and soft tissue envelope is ready.

Subsequently, the patient is brought into the consultation office where the surgeon and the patient evaluate the photos and discuss what can be achieved with surgery based on the patient's examination. In certain patients, the desire for a certain length and counterrotation cannot be achieved due to skin limitations. This discussion ensures that both the surgeon and the patient have similar goals for surgery and that expectations of the patient are managed.

It is important to note that even though lengthening of the nose is desired, it is important to maintain an aesthetic infratip break as well as supratip break.

PROCEDURE
Costal Cartilage Harvest

Cartilage grafting in rhinoplasty can come from several sources, including septal, auricular, and costal. Oftentimes in revision rhinoplasty, there is some septal cartilage remaining inside the nose in order for septal cartilage to be used for cartilage grafting. However, in the overly shortened nose, there is generally the need for stronger and larger amounts of cartilage, which would render the septal cartilage insufficient. Because of the soft nature of auricular cartilage, it is not ideal for structural grafting of the nose. Our preferred source of grafting for revision rhinoplasties is using costal cartilage. Cartilage taken from the rib is both abundant and strong. In the overly shortened nose, there is a deficit of nasal cartilage for tip support, and thus, using costal cartilage is preferred.

For costal cartilage harvest, the incision is marked in either the right-sided inframammary crease in female patients or infrapectoral crease in male patients. This generally translates to either the fifth, sixth, or seventh rib depending on each patient's anatomy, musculature, breast size, or breast implant size. A 1.0-cm to 1.5-cm incision is made, which allows for a very small and hidden incision. In addition, during rib cartilage harvest, a small piece of overlying rib perichondrium is

harvested at the same time, as it can be used later and placed over areas where the skin is thinner to help improve the vascularity of the nasal tip skin and decrease the visibility of cartilage grafts. In general, a 4-cm to 5-cm piece of rib cartilage can be harvested (**Fig. 1**).

Cartilage Grafting

The most important use of cartilage is going to be for a caudal septal extension graft. Not only can a caudal septal extension graft lengthen an overly shorten nose, but it can also help to counterrotate the tip. The graft should be designed to fit each individual depending on the remnant caudal septum. The caudal septal extension graft is generally wider at the top and tapered as it becomes more inferior toward the floor of the nose. In cases in which the caudal septum is just overly short or has been overly shortened and trimmed, a large piece of cartilage can be used to replace the entire caudal septum and act as a wider-based caudal septal extension graft.

The caudal septal extension graft is placed on the end of the septum and must be carefully measured to prevent any overlap of cartilage that can then lead to inadvertent twisting of the tip or widening at the caudal septal region. The caudal septal extension graft can then be fixated by extended spreader grafts or small pieces of septal reinforcement grafts carved from the rib cartilage. For septal cartilage that has significant deviation or memory, additional support can be achieved from polydioxanone plates (0.25 mm and perforated with an 18-gauge needle) sutured to areas of the caudal septum or L-strut or as a small piece of inferior reinforcement in addition to extended spreader grafts. These pieces of cartilage are sutured in placed with 5-0 polydioxanone sutures (PDS). To set the tip projection and rotation, the medial crura can then be sutured onto the caudal septal extension graft once the graft itself has been secured. This can be achieved with a 4-0 plain gut suture through the mucosa and the cartilage to first set the position and then reinforced with 5-0 PDS sutures (**Fig. 2**).

The caudal septal extension graft can also be sutured and fixated to the nasal spine if there is any question of possible deviation of this graft during healing or when the caudal septum inferiorly is quite shortened and additional support is needed. This can be achieved by using a hole puncher to make a hole in the nasal spine and then using a 5-0 PDS to suture the end of the graft to the nasal spine.

Although spreader grafts are usually used for internal nasal valve collapse or any middle vault

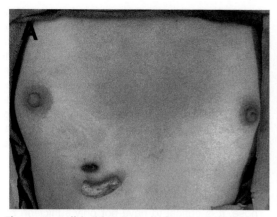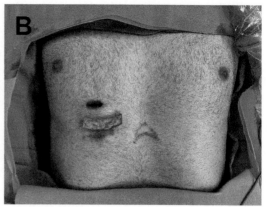

Fig. 1. A small incision is made for rib cartilage harvest usually in the inframammary (*A*) or infrapectoral (*B*) crease.

deficiencies, they can also be used as support for the caudal septal extension graft. By making them longer to extend beyond the caudal septal angle, they can be sutured with 5-0 PDS to fixate to the caudal septal extension graft. This actually reinforces the patient's own L-strut or septum and allows for a better foundation when the nasal skin is healing over the tip. Although this may lead to the sensation of patients feeling that the tip is harder or less mobile than before surgery, this will lead to less deviation and warping of the tip. Over time, the feeling at the nasal tip will also soften.

Depending on the amount of middle vault reinforcement and reconstruction that is needed, rib cartilage can be carved into grafts of different widths, different heights, and different lengths of spreader grafts. It is important to not have the grafts be too thin because it would not offer enough support at the caudal septal extension

graft, and the tip has a higher possibility of twisting to one of the sides, especially when redraping the skin, which applies pressure to the caudal septal extension graft.

Dorsal and Tip Aesthetics

Regardless of the length of the nose and the amount of lengthening that can be or is achieved, the tip aesthetics must be maintained. Tip aesthetics are dependent on both the transition between the dorsum and the tip, also known as the supratip break, as well as the transition from the tip to the medial crural area, known as the infratip break. Because of these relationships, the dorsal height often needs to be adjusted to allow for ideal aesthetics. If there is an insufficient supratip break, it is likely that the caudal dorsum or the length of the entire dorsum needs to be reduced. Although less common, if there is too much of a supratip

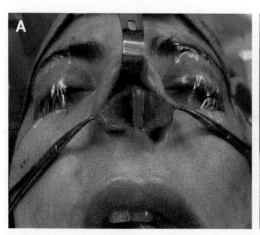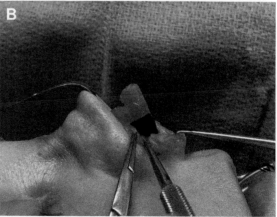

Fig. 2. (*A*) A septal extension graft is sutured in place and is fixated with extended spreader grafts inferiorly. (*B*) Side view of extended spreader sutured to septal extension.

break, there may be a need for dorsal augmentation. Once these components are set, tip grafts and infratip grafts can be used to further modify tip location and aesthetics.

It is also important to note that in individuals with thin or compromised skin, there may be a need for additional camouflage in the area of the tip. Rib perichondrium or deep temporalis fascia are both viable options that can be placed over the area of the tip and sutured in place using a 5-0 chromic suture to prevent migration once the skin soft tissue envelope is closed.

POSTOPERATIVE CARE

At the end of surgery, Doyle splints are generally placed in each nasal cavity and sutured to the caudal septum to prevent any additional swelling or accumulation of blood in between the septal mucosal flaps, especially in the caudal septal region, which can lead to prolonged swelling. A thermal plastic splint or cast is often placed on the nose down toward the supratip area. The tip skin is left exposed so that it can be evaluated for any vascular compromise.

Over the area of the rib cartilage harvest, there is usually a waterproof dressing of Steri Strips (3M, St Paul, MN) and Tegaderm, which allows for the patient to be able to shower during the week.

The patient is discharged after surgery with antibiotics for 1 week, as well as detailed instructions for keeping the incisions clean. The patient is seen on postoperative day 1 to ensure that there is no septal hematoma and to discuss with the patients the results of surgery. The patient's next appointment is on postoperative day 7 during which the Doyle splints as well as the thermoplastic splint is removed. At this appointment, tape is placed over the nasal dorsum to help contain any additional swelling and to ensure that during healing, the skin soft tissue envelope settles down well over the new cartilaginous framework of the nose.

DISCUSSION

For effective lengthening of the overly shortened nose, it is critical to have not only sufficient, but also strong cartilage. This usually requires costal cartilage as there is generally insufficient septal cartilage even without extensive prior septoplasty. By experienced surgeons, costal cartilage can be harvested safely and through a small well-hidden incision with low to no morbidity. The main limitation for the lengthening of the nose is the quality and mobility of the skin soft tissue envelope and adequate evaluation before surgery, as well as discussion with the patient is imperative to achieving desired results and managing patient expectations.

After lengthening is achieved, it is critical that the tip is evaluated as an aesthetic supratip and infratip break are always desired. Grafting at the tip and infratip are finesse techniques that can further modify the tip location.

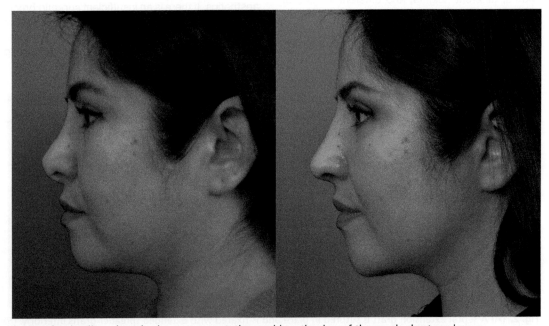

Fig. 3. After healing, there is nice counter rotation and lengthening of the overly shortened nose.

In patients with compromised skin due to multiple previous surgeries or naturally thin skin, it is also important to be able to camouflage the grafting at the tip and rib perichondrium and deep temporalis fascia are 2 options that are easy to obtain (**Fig. 3**).

DISCLOSURE

The authors have nothing to disclose.

REFERENCES

1. Hormozi AK, Toosi AB. Rhinometry: an important clinical index for evaluation of the nose before and after rhinoplasty. Aesthet Plast Surg 2008;32(02):286–93.

2. Toriumi DM, Bared A. Revision of the surgically over-shortened nose. Facial Plast Surg 2012;28:407–16.

3. Naficy S, Baker SR. Lengthening the short nose. Arch Otolaryngol Head Neck Surg 1998;124:809–13.

Management of the Cephalic Positioning of the Lower Lateral Cartilage in Modern Rhinoplasty
An Algorithmic Approach

Behnam Bohluli, DMD, FRCD(C)[a],*, Shahrokh C. Bagheri, DMD, MD[b],
Gholamhosein Adham, DMD[c], Omid Tofighi, DMD[d]

KEYWORDS

• Cephalic positioning • Lateral crural strut • Alar contouring graft • Pseudomalpositioning

KEY POINTS

• Cephalic positioning of lateral cruras literally means that the cartilage does not support the nasal rim.
• Cephalic positioning is a relatively common anatomic variant of lower lateral cartilages that shows an extremely vulnerable rhinoplasty patient.
• In these patients, any reductive technique, such as cephalic trimming without compensation, worsens the situation and may lead to esthetic failures and airway compromise.
• True cephalic malpositioning needs to be diagnosed from pseudomalpositions preoperatively.
• The presence of the pseudomalposition does not mean that it can be ignored. Either malposition or pseudomalposition is best to be diagnosed and considered in the treatment plan.

INTRODUCTION

Cephalic malpositioning of the lower lateral cartilages has been the subject of many longstanding debates in rhinoplasty. In 1978, Sheen[1] stated that lower lateral cartilages in some rhinoplasty patients are not parallel to nostril rims and are rotated toward the septum. He noticed that in this group of patients the nasal tip is flat, broad, and ball shaped, and alar rims have retractions and show a typical parentheses appearance (**Fig. 1**). He called these deformities cephalic malpositioning of the lower lateral cartilages and recommend restoring it by repositioning techniques.

Constantian[2–5] conducted several studies that make up the backbone of the literature on cephalic malpositioning and rhinoplasty. In 1993, he performed a comprehensive analysis on a group of his rhinoplasty patients. He found that, in contrast to original beliefs, cephalic position of the lateral crus was not a rare condition and was detected in 46% of the assessed patients. He demonstrated that alar malposition has a direct effect on external nasal valve function. Surprisingly, he showed that, when the malpositioned lateral cruras are repaired, nasal airflow increases 2 times more than preoperative values.[3]

In 2000, Constantian[4] reviewed 150 secondary rhinoplasty patients to find the main anatomic structures that more commonly lead to revisions and failures of the rhinoplasty. He found that cephalic malpositioning, deep nasal radix/dorsum,

a Oral and Maxillofacial Surgery, University of Toronto, 124 Edward St, Toronto, ON M5G 1G6, Canada;
b Georgia Oral and Facial Reconstructive Surgery, 4561 Olde Perimeter Way, Atlanta, GA 30346, USA;
c private practice, Pouya building, Navab st, Golsar Ave, Rasht, Iran; d private practice, No. 11, 2nd floor, sepehr build.(1425), shariati Av., Gholhak, Tehran, Iran
* Corresponding author.
E-mail address: bbohluli@yahoo.com

Oral Maxillofacial Surg Clin N Am 33 (2021) 131–141
https://doi.org/10.1016/j.coms.2020.09.008

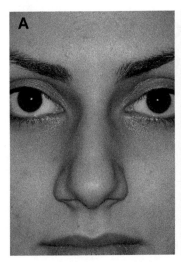
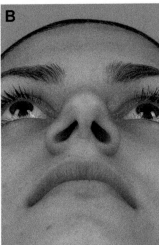

Fig. 1. (*A, B*) Ball-shaped tip, pinched nose, parentheses alar walls indicate cephalic orientation of the lateral crural cartilages.

and low projection of the tip are the main 4 anatomic variations that can end up in unacceptable rhinoplasty outcomes.

These findings are frequently supported in later studies.[6,7] For nearly 2 decades, all efforts were made to find the most effective way to correct the malpositioned cartilage.

One of the first controversies appeared in 2000 when the founder of this concept (Jack Sheen) stated that cephalic malpositioning is not a deformity, and he has not chosen the proper terminology.[8] He proposed that cephalic positioning is a better term that indicates a relatively common anatomic variation of the lower lateral cartilage. He states that he does not necessarily address the issue when parentheses appearance and tip fullness are not the main concerns of the patients, and he plans very conservative treatments, such as tip grafts and alar contouring grafts, instead of major repositioning approaches.[8]

Çakir and colleagues[9–11] demonstrated that in many of the seemingly malpositioned noses, lower lateral cartilages are in the proper position, and the parentheses and ball-tip appearance is due to the length of lateral crura and its configuration. He proposed pseudomalposition to define this group of patients. Daniel and Palhazi[12] showed that some other anatomic configurations might mimic the characteristics of a cephalic position of alar cartilages, and it seems that pseudomalposition may include a greater number of rhinoplasty patients.

Here, the authors give an overview of the current concepts in the diagnosis and management of cephalic positioning of the alar cartilages. The focus is to provide a practical algorithm to differentiate the most common possibilities regarding cephalically positioned cartilage and introduce the predictable approaches for each of them.

DEFINITION OF THE TRUE CEPHALIC POSITION BY ITS RELEVANT ANATOMY

The lower lateral cartilage makes up the framework and supports alar walls and nasal tip. The lower lateral cartilage is usually divided into medial, middle, and lateral crus. The lateral crus runs parallel with the alar rim up to half of the length of the alar wall and then turns cephalically. Therefore, the lower half of the alar wall is devoid of cartilage.[1,13,14] Lateral crural cartilage at its lateral end reaches to the accessory cartilage (**Fig. 2**). A common perichondrium of accessory cartilage and lower lateral cartilage makes up the alar ring.[14]

The long axis of the lower lateral cartilage makes up typically a 45° to the nasal septum, and if it is

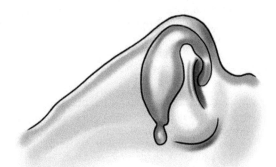

Fig. 2. Caudal edge of the lateral crura parallels the alar rim up to half of its length and then turns cephalically.

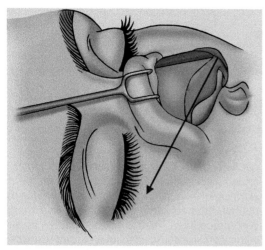

Fig. 3. In usual anatomy, extension of the long axis of the lateral crura reaches the lateral canthus.

extended by an imaginary line, reaches to the lateral canthus of the eye. In cephalic positioning, this angle is more acute and will turn toward the medial canthus of the eye (**Fig. 3**). In original descriptions from Sheen,[1–5] the distance of 7 mm and more from the caudal margin of the cartilage, a border of the alar rim, is the other parameter showing that cartilage is not in the proper position. This anatomic variation means a larger amount of the alar wall is not supported by cartilage, and any reductive procedure may deteriorate the situation in both esthetics and function.

DEFINITION OF THE PSEUDOCEPHALIC POSITION BY ITS RELEVANT ANATOMY

Pseudomalpositioning means that cephalocaudally alar cartilages are in the proper position, but because of their relative angulations to upper lateral cartilages (resting angle) (**Fig. 4**) or their morphologic shapes, they mimic all or some of characteristics of true cephalic positioning.[9–11]

Zelnik and Gingrass[13] did an extensive study on morphology of the lateral crural cartilage. They demonstrated that lateral cartilages do not have a flat surface and may have the 6 main shapes: they may be (1) smooth convex (10%) (**Fig. 5**A), (2) convex anteriorly concave posteriorly (30%) (**Fig. 5**B), (3) concave anteriorly convex posteriorly (25%) (**Fig. 5**C), (4) concave anteriorly and posteriorly (25%) (**Fig. 5**D), and (5) concave (**Fig, 5**E), (6) totally irregular (5%).

Çakir and colleagues[9–11] in 2013 demonstrated that the rotation of the lateral crura along the long axis considerably changes the shape of the nose. They showed that the caudal border of the cartilage is somewhat higher than the cephalic

edge. They introduced the resting angle of the lower lateral cartilage, that is, the angle between lower lateral cartilage and the upper lateral cartilage (see **Fig. 4**). There are few suture techniques to change this angle and correct this type of pseudomalformation.[11,15,16]

The third type of the pseudomalformation is the long lateral crural cartilage. Lateral crural tension suture is an innovative concept that resolves the source of the pathologic condition and easily solves the deformity.[17]

FUNCTIONAL EVALUATION

There are many methods to evaluate and document the function of the external nasal valve. Rhinomanometry, acoustic rhinometry, endoscopic evaluation, and direct visualization with nasal speculum and proper lighting are the methods that are frequently used and provide valuable data.[18] Meanwhile, the forced inspiration test is an easy and practical way that may be done preoperatively or any time in postoperative follow-up. In this test, patient is asked to make a deep inspiration, and the movement of the lateral walls is observed and documented. There may be unilateral, bilateral, partial, or total incompetencies of the external nasal valve (**Fig. 6**). It is recommended to add this test to routine rhinoplasty photography.[1–3,18]

DESCRIPTION OF THE ALGORITHM

The algorithm shown in **Fig. 7** aims to provide a road map for decision-making based on current evidence of rhinoplasty literature.

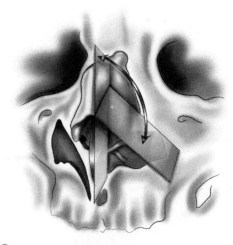

Fig. 4. Improper angle between lateral crural and upper lateral cartilage (rising angle) may mimic the cephalic positioning appearance.

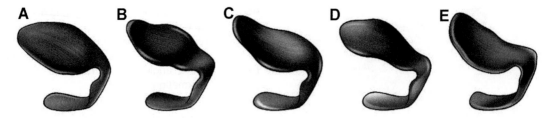

Fig. 5. (*A–E*) Anatomic variations of the lateral crural cartilage.

The first step is to determine the true cephalic position from pseudomalpositioning in suspicious patients (ball shape, broad tip with parentheses appearance of ala). Currently, there are 2 landmarks to detect a true malpositioning. The first one is the long axis of the lateral crural. For inexperienced eyes, cartilage borders can be marked and shaded in life-size photographs. The long axis is drawn to see if it meets lateral canthus or comes closer toward medial canthus. The second hallmark is the distance between the cartilage edge and the alar birder; if it is more than 7 mm, true

cephalic positioning may be confirmed. Then, a forced inspiration test may be performed. If there is no external nasal valve incompetencies, the patient and the surgeon may decide to avoid complex procedures, plan a suboptimal rhinoplasty with minimal reduction techniques, and use tip sutures and grafts and alar rim grafts instead. In the case of nasal valve incompetencies and true cephalic positioning, restoration of cephalic positioning with lateral crural strut would be recommended.

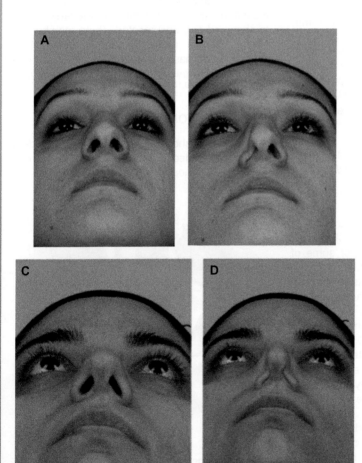

Fig. 6. (*A–D*) Forced inspiration test is an easy way to evaluate and document the function of the external nasal valve. Abstracts: incompetency may be unilateral (*C, D*) or bilateral.

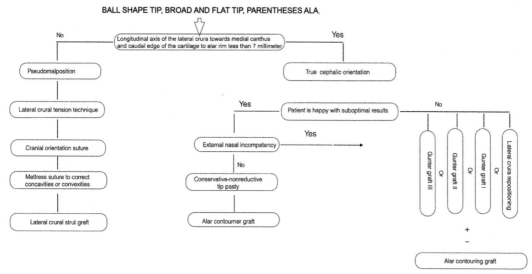

Fig. 7. Diagnosis and management of cephalic positioning.

In the pseudomalposition of the lateral crural cartilage, it is thought that cephalocaudally cartilages are in proper position, but the length of cartilage, angulation of the cartilage, or inherited shape of the cartilage has made the deformity. Many conservative and effective methods are advocated that easily restore the cause of the problem. Here, the authors have suggested detecting the problem and starting from more conservative approaches and to use lateral crural strut when the other methods do not provide an ideal outcome.

TRUE CEPHALIC POSITIONS: CONSERVATIVE APPROACHES TO TRUE CEPHALIC POSITIONING

When the patient is not willing to undergo extensive operations, and more importantly, is satisfied with suboptimal results, conservative methods may be applied.[1] It is recommended to do minimal or no cephalic trim of the lateral cruras. Suturing techniques may help to flatten the cartilage and improve the shape of the cartilage.[17] Although it cannot improve real cephalic orientation of the cartilage, alar rim graft is an effective adjunctive technique that reinforces the rim and improves parentheses appearance and is recommended in this group of the patients (**Fig. 8**).

ALAR CONTOURING GRAFT

Alar contouring graft has originally been described by Troell and colleagues[19] to reinforce weak external nasal valves. Meanwhile, later studies showed more potentials of this technique.[20–23]

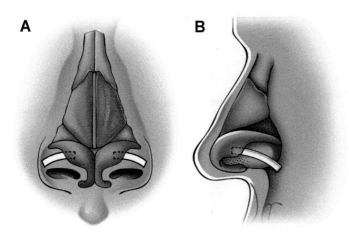

A **B**

Fig. 8. (*A, B*) Alar contouring graft is an effective and simple way to correct true malpositioning when extensive surgery is not planned.

Alar contouring graft is a narrow strip of the cartilage, placed in the margin of the alar wall (**Fig. 9**).

The main indications for this graft are reinforcement of the external nasal valve, correction of the alar retraction, and restoration of the soft triangle deformity. This technique is frequently used in both primary and secondary rhinoplasties.[20,22,23]

TECHNIQUE

- By using delicate converse scissors, a narrow subcutaneous pocket is created in the caudal margin of the alar rim (see **Fig. 6**A).
- A thin strip of cartilage (10–15 mm length, 1–3 mm width) is prepared.
- The graft is inserted inside the pocket (see **Fig. 6**B).
- The tip of the graft may be shortened, morselized, crushed, or tailored depending on the need and indication.

PEARLS AND PITFALLS

- Alar contouring graft may be prepared from septal, conchal, or rib cartilage.
- Alar contouring graft is a nonanatomic graft (is to be placed in a location that is not normally filled by cartilage). Therefore, like the other nonanatomic grafts, sharp edges of the graft

are best to be morselized or tailored to avoid irregularities and visible edges on the skin.
- Alar contouring graft is quite useful in mild to moderate deformities. In the case of severe scarring in revision patients or severe alar retractions, a more complex plan, such as composite conchal graft, may be indicated.

DEFINITIVE APPROACHES TO TRUE CEPHALIC POSITIONING

Lateral crural repositioning and lateral crural struts are the mainstays of the treatment of true cephalic orientations.

LATERAL CRURAL REPOSITIONING

This technique was first introduced in 1993 by Hamra.[24] It is an effective method to repair cephalic-positioned lateral crural cartilage. This method may be applied in both open and closed approaches.[24–26]

TECHNIQUES

- Adequate infiltration of local anesthesia is used beneath lateral crural cartilage for easier dissection.
- Lateral crural cartilage is dissected away from its underlying skin (**Fig. 10**C, D).

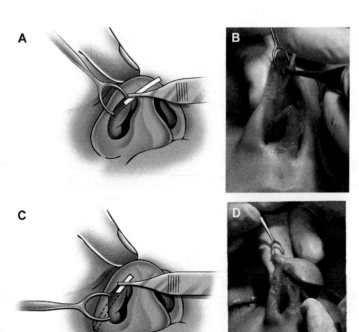

Fig. 9. (*A–D*) Alar contouring graft (alar rim graft) is a thin rectangular piece of the cartilage that is placed in a snug pocket in the alar rim.

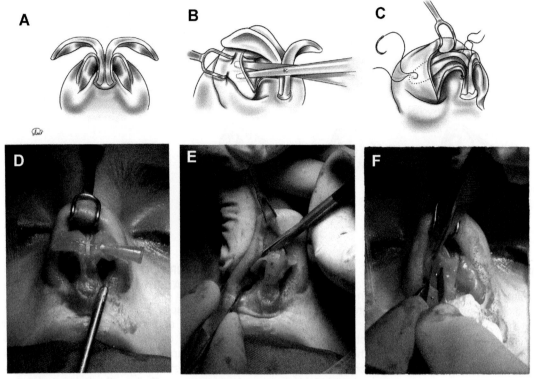

Fig. 10. (*A–F*) Lateral crural repositioning to repair lateral crural malpositioning.

- A pocket is created in the lobule area (the soft tissue caudal to the infracartilagenous incision) (**Fig. 10**B, E).
- The lateral crura is inserted in the pocket and fixed with a few stitches (**Fig. 10**C, F).

PEARLS AND PITFALLS

- Lateral crural repositioning is rarely used alone, and it is commonly combined with one of the modifications of the lateral strut graft.
- This procedure needs a precise technique to obtain symmetric results.

LATERAL CRURAL STRUT (GUNTER GRAFT)

Lateral crural strut is a strong tool in modern rhinoplasty. As per original descriptions of technique by Gunter and Friedman,[26] this technique is effective in repairing cephalic positioning, shaping the lateral crus, correction of alar retraction, and reinforcement external airway.[27,28] In this technique, a quadrangular piece of cartilage graft is fixed underneath the lateral crus.[12,27,28] Based on the needs and indications, different sizes of the graft in different modifications (types) may be used[12] (**Fig.11**A–F). **Table 1** shows different types of the lateral crural strut graft and their indications.

TECHNIQUE

- Adequate infiltration is applied of local anesthetic on the vestibular skin for easier dissection of the underlying skin.
- The skin underlying the lateral crural cartilage is dissected from the dome area toward the accessory cartilage.
- A rectangular piece of septal cartilage (3–5 mm in 10–15 mm) is prepared.
- Cartilages are placed and fixed under the surface of the lateral cartilage.
- Based on the type of the graft to be used (see **Fig. 11**; **Table 1**), dissection and graft placement may be extended to the alar rim, accessory cartilages, and basal wall soft tissues.

PEARLS AND PITFALLS

- Lateral crural strut graft needs a precise technique to achieve the optimal outcome and to avoid asymmetries.
- Septal cartilage is the choice for this graft. However, conchal cartilage and rib cartilage may be used for this purpose.
- Alar contouring graft may be added if the effects of the Gunter graft seem to be inadequate.

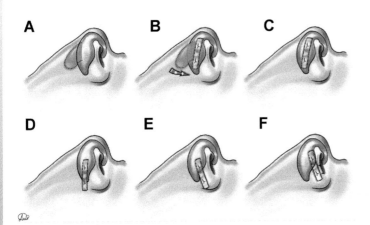

Fig. 11. Different methods to correct true malpositioning, from repositioning to different types of the Gunter graft.

PSEUDOMALPOSITION

Treatment of pseudomalposition is based on finding the source of the deformity. If it is due to lateral crural length (excessive length), lateral crural tension sutures may effectively solve the problem. Therefore, in the authors' algorithm, they start with lateral crural tensioning. This technique is a routine step in many modern rhinoplasty procedures. It is very conservative and reproducible. It is shown that, in most pseudomalpositions, the problem is solved in the most cases. Whereas, when there is an inherent malformation in lateral crural cartilages (concavities and convexities), mattress sutures are ideal options. Finally, when the problem is axial orientation of the lateral crus, related mattress sutures would be recommended.

The last modality in the management of the pseudomalposition would be lateral crural strut. Lateral crural strut is a reliable tool that may be applied when other options do not provide optimal outcomes.

LATERAL CRURAL TENSION SUTURE (MODIFIED LATERAL STEAL SUTURE)

The idea of shaping the nasal cartilages by sutures was invented and popularized by Tebbetts in 1994.[28] Later on, various suturing techniques with different applications were introduced. Kridel and colleagues[29] (1989) presented an innovative suture technique. Their method aims to increase tip projection and nasolabial angle by borrowing (stealing) a few millimeters of the long lateral crura to medial crura. The technique was very conservative and relatively simple compared with other available modalities. Davis (2015) and Çakir (2016) made a significant improvement to the concept. They showed that in many patients, lateral crus is longer than its soft tissue envelope, which may cause buckling and distortion of the cartilage. It causes tip malformation and airway damage.[9,30] Lateral crural steal transfers extra length and can easily restore these deformations by making a strong flat lateral crus.[30,31] Davis

Table 1
Different types of the lateral crural strut graft (Gunter graft) and their indications

LCS Types	Specifications of the Graft	Indication
Conventional GUNTER GRAFT	The graft does not exceed the borders of lateral crural cartilage	To shape the lateral crus
GUNTER + TRANSPOSITION	The graft does not exceed the borders of lateral crural cartilage	To repair malposition
GUNTER I	The graft extends to undersurface of accessory cartilages	To shape lateral crus
GUNTER II	The graft extends to alar base	To repair cephalic orientation
GUNTER III	The graft is extended to alar rim	To correct alar retractions

proposed stabilizing this new tip to a strong septal extension graft.[30] These changes resulted in the advent of lateral crural tension suture in modern rhinoplasty.

MATTRESS SUTURE

Gruber and colleagues[32] proposed simple mattress sutures to restore concavities and convexities of the lateral crural cartilage. This technique is quite conservative and reproducible, so it may be used as an option in correcting lateral crus deformities before proceeding with more sophisticated approaches.[15,32]

The technique to correct a convexity is as follows:

- Adequate local anesthetic is infiltrated on vestibular skin to make the pass of needle easier.
- The needle enters perpendicular to the long axis of the lateral crural cartilage, and with the same pass, comes out about 5 mm from the entering point. The second pass is made at about 5 mm to the first pass (**Fig. 12**).
- By tightening the tie, the convexity is flattened, and when the ideal form is achieved, several knots are added.[15,32]

The technique to correct a concavity is as follows:

- Adequate local anesthetic is infiltrated on vestibular skin to make the pass of the needle easier.
- A needle enters parallel to the long axis of the lateral crural cartilage (the opposite direction

compared with convexity deformity) and, with the same pass, comes out about 5 mm from the entering point. The second pass is made at about 5 mm to the first pass (**Fig. 13**).
- By tightening the tie, the concavity is flattened, and when the ideal form is achieved, several knots are added.

PEARLS AND PITFALLS

- This technique has a steep learning curve. Therefore, the first trials may need several redos and adjustments.
- Extremely wide and narrow lateral crura are not good choices for this technique.
- Small bites may have suboptimal effects, whereas very large bites may distort the cartilage.
- Two or 3 mattress sutures may be applied next to each other to correct a deformity.
- The needle is passed between cartilage and underlying skin. Care should be taken not to pass through the underlying skin.
- PDS or Vycril 5-0 is the recommended suture material for this purpose.

CRANIAL REORIENTING SUTURES

Several investigators have emphasized the importance of the axial orientation of the lateral crus.[11,15,16] Typically, the caudal edge of the lateral crura is somewhat superior to the cephalic

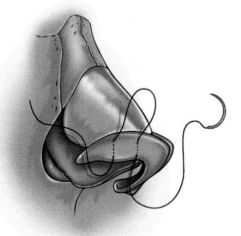

Fig. 12. Mattress suture to correct convexity.

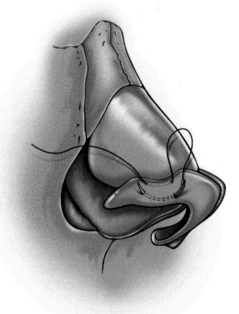

Fig. 13. Mattress suture to correct concavity.

edge of the cartilage.[11,15] The angle between the lower lateral and upper lateral cartilage is to be around 110.[9–11] Wider angle means the caudal edge is at the level of cephalic edge or even inferior to it. This orientation makes a ball-shaped tip and parentheses rims (pseudomalposition).[9–11] Cranial orientation suture has been introduced with different names and technical details. However, in general, it is a simple mattress suture to evert cranial edge of the cartilage and turn the cartilage along its long axis.[15]

PEARLS AND PITFALLS

- Cranial orientation suture is to be the last step in tip plasty.
- Preprocedure marking and precise method are needed to avoid asymmetries.

LATERAL CRURAL STRUT GRAFT

A classic lateral crural strut graft is an efficient method to shape the lateral crural cartilage and correct concavities and convexities of the lateral crus. Meanwhile, in contrast to true malpositions, if there is no structural deficiency and more conservative methods work, it may be the last option.

SUMMARY

Cephalic positioning has been an extremely controversial issue in rhinoplasty. Although many investigators now use it as a prevalent anatomic variation and recommend a comprehensive treatment plan to solve it, some others believe cephalic positioning is overstated, and many of the diagnosed cases are pseudomalpositions. This review shows that either true cephalic positioning or pseudomalpositionings show a vulnerable rhinoplasty patient. In fact, it is a red flag that shows routine reductive rhinoplasty techniques may end up in sever functional and aesthetic complications. The authors suggest an easy algorithm to help in the process of decision-making. If because of any reason the cosmetic surgeon and the patient plan to avoid a wider procedure, it is best practice to plan minimum changes and avoid aggressive reductive techniques. The other dominant factor is external nasal incompetency that is very common in these patients. It is clear that the nasal airway cannot be underestimated. Therefore, in the case of valve incompetencies, reinforcement techniques may be mandatory, and conservative noninvasive approaches may not be an option; it may be better to decline an aesthetic nose surgery when the demands and possible results do not match.

CLINICS CARE POINTS

- Cephalic positioning of the lateral cruras is best to be diagnosed preoperatively.
- Ball-shaped tip, parenthesis nasal walls, and weak external nasal valves are the main indicators of the lateral crural malpositioning.
- Reductive techniques may end in sever functional and esthetic complications.
- Pseudomal positions may be corrected by conservative approaches.

DISCLOSURE

The authors have nothing to disclose.

REFERENCES

1. Sheen JH. Aesthetic rhinoplasty. St Louis (MO): CV Mosby; 1978.
2. Constantian MB. Functional effects of alar cartilage malposition. Ann Plast Surg 1993;30(6):487–99.
3. Constantian MB. The incompetent external nasal valve: pathophysiology and treatment in primary and secondary rhinoplasty. Plast Reconstr Surg 1994;93(5):919–31 [discussion: 932–3].
4. Constantian MB. Four common anatomic variants that predispose to unfavorable rhinoplasty results: a study based on 150 consecutive secondary rhinoplasties. Plast Reconstr Surg 2000;105(1):316–31 [discussion: 332–3].
5. Constantian MB. The two essential elements for planning tip surgery in primary and secondary rhinoplasty: observations based on review of 100 consecutive patients. Plast Reconstr Surg 2004;114(6):1571–81 [discussion: 1582–5]. Review.
6. Silva EN. The relation between the lower lateral cartilages and the function of the external nasal valve. Aesthet Plast Surg 2019;43(1):175–83.
7. Sepehr A, Alexander AJ, Chauhan N, et al. Cephalic positioning of the lateral crura: implications for nasal tip-plasty. Arch Facial Plast Surg 2010;12(6):379–84.
8. Sheen JH. Rhinoplasty: personal evolution and milestones. Plast Reconstr Surg 2000;105(5):1820–52 [discussion: 1853].
9. Çakır B, Öreroğlu AR, Daniel RK. Surface aesthetics and analysis. Clin Plast Surg 2016;43(1):1–15.
10. Çakır B, Öreroğlu AR, Daniel RK. Surface aesthetics in tip rhinoplasty: a step-by-step guide. Aesthet Surg J 2014;34(6):941–55.
11. Çakir B, Doğan T, Öreroğlu AR, et al. Rhinoplasty: surface aesthetics and surgical techniques. Aesthet Surg J 2013;33(3):363–75.
12. Daniel RK, Palhazi P. Osseocartilaginous vault. In: Daniel RK, Palhazi P, editors. Rhinoplasty: an anatomical and clinical atlas. New York: Springer; 2018. p. 113–63.

13. Zelnik J, Gingrass RP. Anatomy of the alar cartilage. Plast Reconstr Surg 1979;64(5):650–3.

14. Daniel RK, Palhazi P, Gerbault O, et al. Rhinoplasty: the lateral crura-alar ring. Aesthet Surg J 2014;34(4): 526–37.

15. Kovacevic M, Wurm J. Cranial tip suture in nasal tip contouring. Facial Plast Surg 2014;30(6):681–7.

16. Toriumi DM. Nasal tip contouring: anatomic basis for management. Facial Plast Surg Aesthet Med 2020; 22(1):10–24.

17. Davis RE. Lateral crural tensioning for refinement of the wide and underprojected nasal tip: rethinking the lateral crural steal. Facial Plast Surg Clin North Am 2015;23(1):23–53.

18. Troell RJ, Powell NB, Riley RW, et al. Evaluation of a new procedure for nasal alar rim and valve collapse: nasal alar rim reconstruction. Otolaryngol Head Neck Surg 2000;122(2):204–11.

19. Unger JG, Roostaeian J, Small KH, et al. Alar contour grafts in rhinoplasty: a safe and reproducible way to refine alar contour aesthetics. Plast Reconstr Surg 2016;137(1):52–61.

20. Kemaloğlu CA, Altıparmak M. The alar rim flap: a novel technique to manage malpositioned lateral crura. Aesthet Surg J 2015;35(8):920–6.

21. Guyuron B, Bigdeli Y, Sajjadian A. Dynamics of the alar rim graft. Plast Reconstr Surg 2015;135(4): 981–6.

22. Gruber RP, Fox P, Peled A, et al. Grafting the alar rim: application as anatomical graft. Plast Reconstr Surg 2014;134(6):880e–7e.

23. Hamra ST. Repositioning the lateral alar crus. Plast Reconstr Surg 1993;92(7):1244–53.

24. Toriumi DM, Asher SA. Lateral crural repositioning for treatment of cephalic malposition. Facial Plast Surg Clin North Am 2015;23(1):55–71.

25. Bared A, Rashan A, Caughlin BP, et al. Lower lateral cartilage repositioning: objective analysis using 3-dimensional imaging. JAMA Facial Plast Surg 2014;16(4):261–7.

26. Gunter JP, Friedman RM. Lateral crural strut graft: technique and clinical applications in rhinoplasty. Plast Reconstr Surg 1997;99(4):943–52.

27. de Oliveira Silva Filho R, Diniz de Pochat V. Anatomical study of the lateral crural strut graft in rhinoplasty and its clinical application. Aesthet Surg J 2016;36(Issue 8):877–83.

28. Tebbetts JB. Shaping and position the nasal tip without structural disruption: a new, systematic approach. Plast Reconstr Surg 1994;94:61–77.

29. Kridel RW, Konior RJ, Shumrick KA, et al. Advances in nasal tip surgery. The lateral crural steal. Arch Otolaryngol Head Neck Surg 1989;115(10):1206–12.

30. Foulad A, Volgger V, Wong B. Lateral crural tensioning for refinement of the nasal tip and increasing alar stability: a case series. Facial Plast Surg 2017;33(3):316–23.

31. Gruber RP, Nahai F, Bogdan MA, et al. Changing the convexity and concavity of nasal cartilages and cartilage grafts with horizontal mattress sutures: part I. Experimental results. Plast Reconstr Surg 2005;115(2):589–94.

32. Gruber RP, Nahai F, Bogdan MA, et al. Changing the convexity and concavity of nasal cartilages and cartilage grafts with horizontal mattress sutures: part II. Clinical results. Plast Reconstr Surg 2005; 115(2):595–606 [discussion: 607–8].

Challenging Rhinoplasty for the Cleft Lip and Palate Patient

Angelo Cuzalina, MD, DDS*, Pasquale G. Tolomeo, MD, DDS

KEYWORDS

- Cleft rhinoplasty • Unilateral/bilateral cleft rhinoplasty • Definitive rhinoplasty • Nasal revision

KEY POINTS

- Secondary (definitive) rhinoplasty is a complex surgical procedure due to the need for multiple surgical stages while dealing with aberrant anatomy.
- Septal extension grafts are constructed from the interior aspect of the rib cartilage, while batten grafts are constructed from the curved portion.
- Application of piriform rim/premaxilla grafts address asymmetry along the midface.
- The use of adjuvant therapies (synthetic fillers and autologous fat grafting) may improve the overall result of the rhinoplasty.
- The surgeon must be able to utilize multiple treatment modalities to address the cleft patient and minimize relapse.

INTRODUCTION

Situated at the middle third of the face, the nose is one of the most common facial structures that is first identified by individuals. Any minute changes are easily identified and are unforgiving. Rhinoplasty is an incredibly intricate surgical procedure, as it involves manipulation of multiple parts, including the skin, cartilage, and bone. Cleft lip and palate patients pose a greater dilemma to the surgeon because of the presence of significant asymmetry and deficiency of underlying tissue and bone. Multiple rhinoplasties may be required in order to achieve esthetic results. The aim of this article is to discuss the secondary (definitive) rhinoplasty as well as adjuvant techniques when treating cleft lip and palate patients.

ANATOMY
Unilateral Cleft and Acquired Nasal Deformity

In the presence of a unilateral cleft, the insertion points of the orbicularis oris are disrupted. On the noncleft side, the orbicularis oris muscle attaches to the ipsilateral aspect of the columella and forces the premaxilla, columella, and caudal nasal septum toward the unaffected side.[1,2] On the cleft side, the orbicularis oris inserts into the ipsilateral alar base and pulls the base laterally, inferiorly, and posteriorly.[1,2] The lower lateral cartilage (LLC) of the cleft side is commonly malformed and contributes to the nasal deformity, creating a more blunted contour[1] (**Fig. 1**). The nostril on the cleft side is significantly wider than the unaffected side and laterally positioned to the affected side because of a blunted medial crus and an elongated lateral crus[1,2] (**Fig. 2**). It is important to note that as the caudal septum deviates toward the unaffected side, the remaining septum deviates toward the cleft side. The presence of septal deviation and decreased nasal aperture leads to an increase in nasal obstruction. Internal vestibular webbing along the nostril margin of the cleft side causes an inward displacement of the margin.[2] The LLC is rotated inward leading to additional nasal obstruction because of a collapse of the external nasal valve; the position of the LLC

Tulsa Surgical Arts, 7322 East 91st Street Tulsa, OK 74133, USA
* Corresponding author.
E-mail address: angelo@tulsasurgicalarts.com

Oral Maxillofacial Surg Clin N Am 33 (2021) 143–159
https://doi.org/10.1016/j.coms.2020.09.012
1042-3699/21/Published by Elsevier Inc.

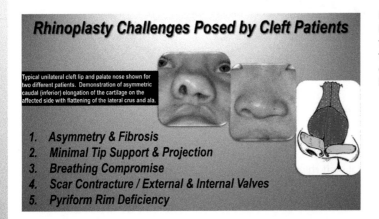

Fig. 1. Surgical challenges presented by cleft lip and palate patients. Malformation of the LLC is present on the cleft side and contributes to the deformity of the nasal tip, creating a blunted contour.

creates a thicker and hooded appearance of the nasal ala.[1] The internal rotation of the LLC is due to excess force from the aberrant position of the alar base and columella, forcing the cartilage posteriorly and inferiorly[3] (**Fig. 3**). LLC asymmetry and septal deviation require surgical intervention that includes an asymmetric lateral crura steal technique in addition to placement of a septal extension graft (SEG; **Figs. 4** and **5**).

Bilateral Cleft and Acquired Nasal Deformity

Bilateral and unilateral nasal cleft deformities share many characteristics, yet bilateral nasal cleft deformities tend to be more symmetric.[1,2] A significant finding in these patients is the presence of a bilateral hypoplastic maxilla with no development of the nasal floor.[2] The alar base is positioned caudally and laterally with significant widening noted. The nasal tip has decreased projection and contour because of the elongation of the lateral crus and shortening of the medial crus[1,2] (**Fig. 6**). The presence of vestibular webbing is noted bilaterally.[2] The nasal septum is usually midline and contributes to the symmetric appearance of the nose. Alternatively, in asymmetry cases, the less affected side creates a pulling force on the septum, resulting in septal deviation to the ipsilateral side.[1,2]

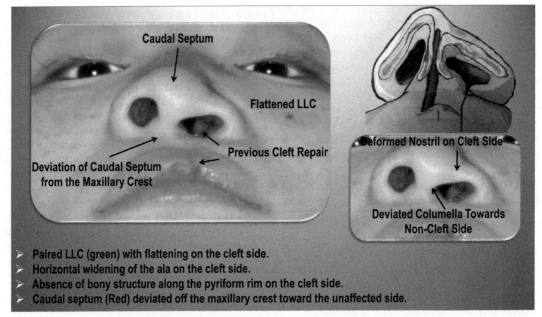

> ➤ Paired LLC (green) with flattening on the cleft side.
> ➤ Horizontal widening of the ala on the cleft side.
> ➤ Absence of bony structure along the pyriform rim on the cleft side.
> ➤ Caudal septum (Red) deviated off the maxillary crest toward the unaffected side.

Fig. 2. Anatomic deviations in cleft lip and palate patients. These patients present with flattening of the LLC on the cleft side, deviation of the caudal septum and columella, alar widening, and absence of bony structures.

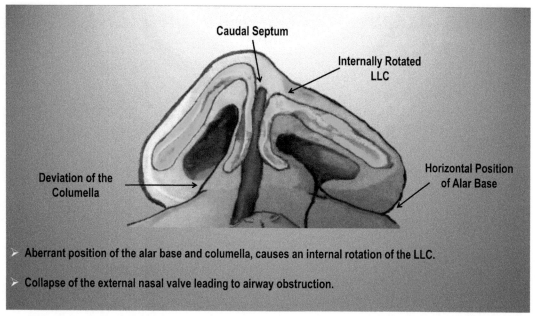

Caudal Septum

Internally Rotated LLC

Deviation of the Columella

Horizontal Position of Alar Base

➤ Aberrant position of the alar base and columella, causes an internal rotation of the LLC.

➤ Collapse of the external nasal valve leading to airway obstruction.

Fig. 3. Internal rotation of the LLC due to the position of the alar base and columella. This internal rotation causes significant airway obstruction.

Surgical Timing

Surgical repair of a cleft nasal deformity is usually performed in multiple stages based on surgical timing: primary, intermediate, and secondary. These patients undergo cleft lip repair with simultaneous primary rhinoplasty around the age of 2 to 3 months.[3–6] Current treatment guidelines recommend surgical intervention at 3 months of age to decrease the risk of surgical and anesthetic complications.[6] An intermediate rhinoplasty is performed during the ages of 5 to 11 years, most commonly at ages 4 to 6 years, before school enrollment.[1,4] The timing of the secondary

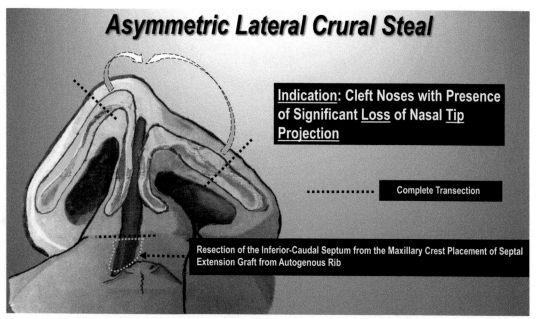

Asymmetric Lateral Crural Steal

Indication: Cleft Noses with Presence of Significant <u>Loss</u> of Nasal <u>Tip</u> Projection

••••••••••• Complete Transection

Resection of the Inferior-Caudal Septum from the Maxillary Crest Placement of Septal Extension Graft from Autogenous Rib

Fig. 4. The authors modified the LCS technique to achieve symmetry in the unilateral cleft as well as increase overall tip projection.

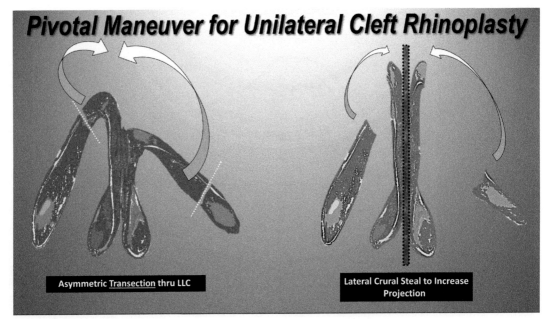

Pivotal Maneuver for Unilateral Cleft Rhinoplasty

Asymmetric <u>Transection</u> thru LLC

Lateral Crural Steal to Increase Projection

Fig. 5. The asymmetric transection of the LLC and the proposed arc of rotation.

(definitive) rhinoplasty depends on the completion of facial growth and maturation, which varies between the genders.[1] Facial maturation occurs between the ages of 14 and 16 years in girls and 16 to 18 years in boys.[1] Additional factors that influence timing of definitive rhinoplasty include patient's size, extent of deformity, and nose size.[5]

Primary Rhinoplasty

Rhinoplasty performed at this stage alone is currently accepted as definitive surgical treatment by many surgeons.[3] It is even considered the standard of care in the United States among other countries.[7] The original notion that primary rhinoplasty can interfere with facial growth has been

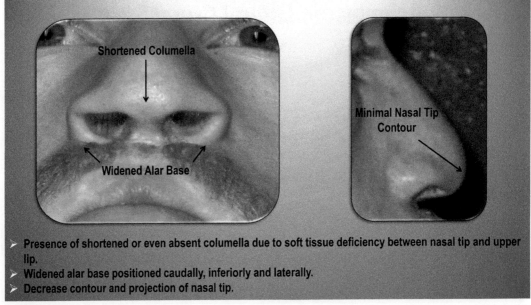

Shortened Columella

Widened Alar Base

Minimal Nasal Tip Contour

➢ Presence of shortened or even absent columella due to soft tissue deficiency between nasal tip and upper lip.
➢ Widened alar base positioned caudally, inferiorly and laterally.
➢ Decrease contour and projection of nasal tip.

Fig. 6. Bilateral cleft lip and palate patients present with a shortened columella with symmetric widening of the alar base and minimal nasal tip contour due to a soft tissue deficiency.

disputed by many recent studies.[1] The primary target of this surgery is to obtain a symmetric nasal tip and alar base.[3] There are many described techniques to correct the asymmetrical unilateral nasal deformity, most notably, the V-Y-Z plasty.[1,8] In general, the LLC is released and repositioned.[1–3,5] The alar base is separated from the pyriform aperture and maxilla to be repositioned symmetrically.[3,5] Nasal tip plasty is performed to enhance its projection.[3] Moreover, the caudal nasal septum is repaired at this stage by attaching it to the anterior nasal spine.[1] The use of a presurgical nasoalveolar molding device can be successful in shaping nasal cartilage within the first 6 weeks after birth, when the cartilage is more elastic because of high levels of circulating maternal estrogen.[9]

Intermediate Rhinoplasty

This surgery is only performed when necessary. Some bilateral cleft nasal deformity patients undergo surgery at this stage to correct a severely asymmetrical nasal tip that was not repaired in primary rhinoplasty.[1,5] In addition, it aims at lengthening a shortened columella.[5] For unilateral nasal deformities, it addresses any residual defects in LLC and lateral vestibular webbing. Septal repositioning and cartilage grafting are not performed at this stage; they are postponed until complete skeletal growth is achieved in adulthood.[1]

Secondary/Definitive

Secondary/definitive intervention is usually required to correct secondary deformities and scarring that develop after primary cleft lip and nose repair. The success of primary rhinoplasty and the severity of secondary deformities are dependent on the surgeon's skill and experience.[7] An open approach is the most common technique used in definitive rhinoplasty, as it allows for enhanced exposure of muscle structure, cartilage, vestibular lining, and dense scarring.[1,3,5] It also aids in precise positioning of the lateral lower cartilage, nasal base, and septum, as well as accurate grafting and suturing.[5]

Goals of definitive rhinoplasty include nasal tip definition, removal of scar and fibrofatty tissue, and nasal obstruction repair (**Fig. 7**).[10,11] In some cases, depending on the complexity of the cleft lip and palate deformity, a Le Fort procedure may be indicated to correct secondary maxillary hypoplasia.[12] Definitive rhinoplasty is typically performed after repairing major skeletal defects with necessary orthognathic surgery.[2]

Incision

Secondary cleft rhinoplasty is almost always performed via an open approach, giving access to different parts of the nose that need reconstruction along with direct visualization. The

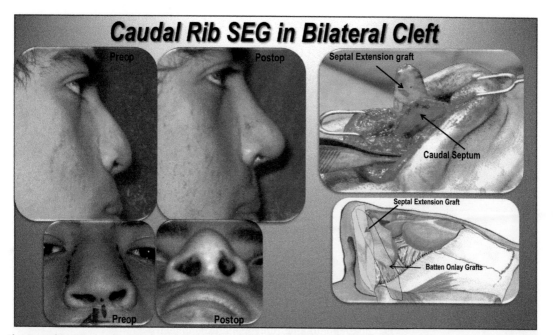

Fig. 7. A shortened columella is commonly seen in bilateral cleft cases due to the lack of soft tissue between the nasal tip and upper lip. These patients require a large and durable SEG harvested from a rib graft in order to overcome fibrosis and increase nasal tip projection. Postop, postoperative; preop, preoperative.

transcolumellar open incision is the most common access technique in definitive rhinoplasty, as it provides better exposure of the septal cartilage as well as the underlying bony and soft tissue structures.[13] The incision is V- or W-shaped and is infracartilaginous. The incision is placed anterior to the footplate segments of the medial crura of the LLC.[13] It is important to note that the medial crura are directly under the skin in the lateral portion of the columella; a superficial dissection is advisable in this area.[1] A medial marginal columella incision is made approximately 1 to 2 mm from the columella edge and extends up to the domal recess. Once the skin flap is elevated, the cartilage and bone components can be examined thoroughly.

Septum

A deviated septum in cleft patients may lead to airway obstruction by way of physical stenosis and turbulent airflow.[14] Correcting the septum involves resecting its cartilaginous and bony parts, including the vomer and perpendicular plate of the ethmoid bone.[14] Simultaneously, it is best to maintain at least 1-cm width of dorsal and caudal septal segments, or L-strut, to preserve the tip and dorsal nasal support.[15,16] There should also be more than 40% fixation area, or contact point, between the nasal crest of the maxilla and L-strut when resecting the caudal septum.[1] The contact point decreases the strain energy and stress values on the septum and relieves excessive load forces on the L-strut, thereby reducing the chances of future nasal deformities, such as a collapse of the dorsal septum or saddle deformity, and nasal tip ptosis.[15] However, in some cases, the septal deviation is severe enough that the resection of the deviated segment and its replacement with a straight graft is necessary. The graft is obtained from septal cartilage, or the rib cartilage may be used if a larger segment is needed.[17] Sutures through the upper lateral cartilages and septum are placed to apply force in the opposite direction of the L-strut deviation, thus correcting it and creating symmetry[18] (**Fig. 8**). In certain cases, a notch is created in the nasal spine using a straight osteotome to allow for a stronger attachment of the caudal strut.[19] Spreader grafts and batten onlay grafts may be harvested from the resected parts of the quadrangular septal cartilage, but most often are obtained from the curved portion of the right sixth rib in order to have adequate shape, size, and strength of cartilage required in the cleft rhinoplasty.[2] A mucoperichondrial flap is raised with caution not to perforate the surrounding mucosa and to allow excellent coverage of a large SEG from rib.[2]

Spreader Graft

Spreader grafts, mainly for the middle third of the nose, are used to open up the internal nasal valve

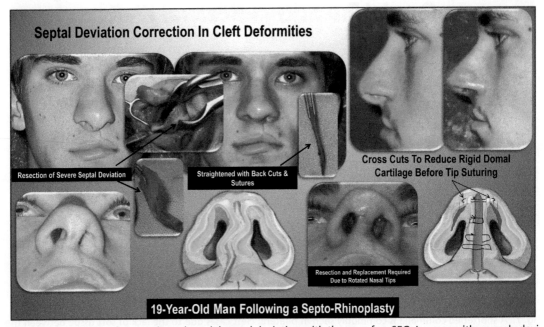

Fig. 8. The correction of severe tip and caudal septal deviation with the use of an SEG. In cases with severely deviated septal cartilage, the cartilage must be resected and grafted.

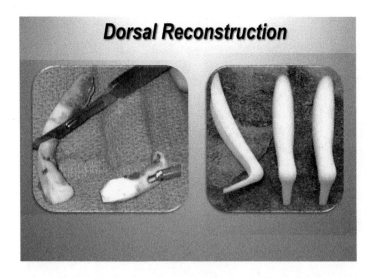

Dorsal Reconstruction

Fig. 9. Options for dorsal reconstruction include autogenous rib graft and silicone implants.

and hence improve breathing.[2,14] They are harvested from either the nasal septal cartilage or part of the harvested rib cartilage. They are placed between the septum and upper lateral cartilage bilaterally and fixated with sutures.[14] If required, the spreader graft can extend more caudally and act as a strut graft for better nasal tip support as well as aiding with septum stability and straightening. Spreader grafts can sometimes be used to correct severe septal deviation by placing the grafts along the dorsal septum, while reattaching the caudal strut to the nasal spine between the medial crura by suture fixation.

Nasal Dorsum and Nasal Bone Osteotomies

The nasal dorsum in cleft patients is most often deficient and less pronounced when compared with that of noncleft patients. This defect is treated with either a silicone implant (Implantech, Ventura, California) or a dorsal onlay rib graft (**Fig. 9**). The septum and nasal bones tend to deviate toward the unaffected side, whereas the base of the nasal dorsum is deviated toward the cleft side.[1] The presence of a prominent dorsal hump requires excision of the cartilaginous base as well as reduction of the bony component using a rasp or

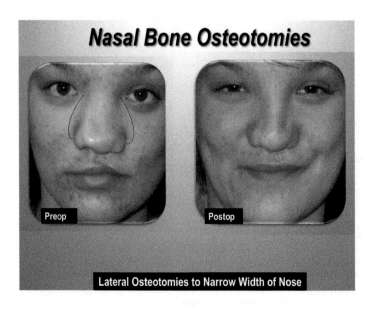

Nasal Bone Osteotomies

Preop   Postop

Lateral Osteotomies to Narrow Width of Nose

Fig. 10. Nasal bone osteotomies are performed to decrease the nasal width and treat an open roof deformity. This is performed by using nasal osteotomes to create micropunctures along the lateral nasal bones followed by in fracturing of the nasal bones.

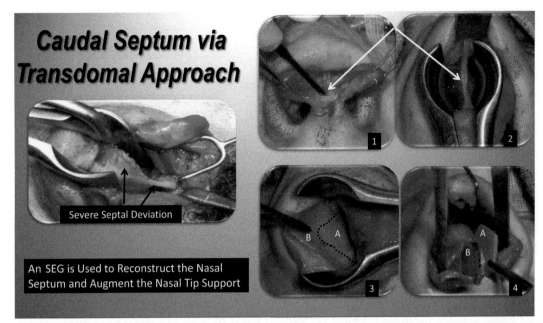

Caudal Septum via Transdomal Approach

Severe Septal Deviation

An SEG is Used to Reconstruct the Nasal Septum and Augment the Nasal Tip Support

Fig. 11. (1) The septum is initially accessed via a transcolumellar incision followed by a transdomal dissection. (2) Dissection along the caudal septal is continued until the septum is exposed down to the anterior nasal spine. (3) It is important to preserve ample caudal septum to allow fixation of the SEG. (A) Planned septal harvest, (B) caudal septum. (4) Fixation of SEG to the caudal septum. The SEG significantly improves nasal tip projection and support even after major amounts of deviated septal cartilage is resected. (A) SEG; (B) native caudal septum.

surgical handpiece. It is important to note that reduction of the dorsal hump will create an open roof deformity that must be addressed. Lateral nasal osteotomies are performed to decrease the width of the nasal bone base as well as treat the open roof deformity. The osteotomies are performed by using a 2- to 3-mm osteotome and creating micropunctures along the planned osteotomies. The osteotome is placed subperiosteal and is guided from a low to high direction,

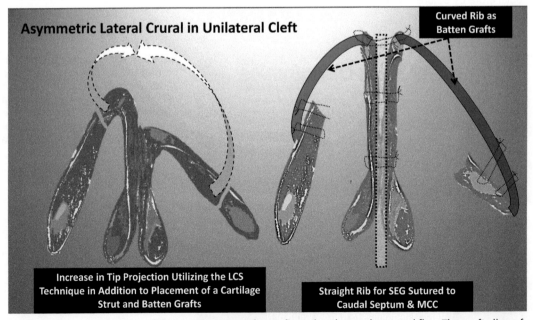

Asymmetric Lateral Crural in Unilateral Cleft

Curved Rib as Batten Grafts

Increase in Tip Projection Utilizing the LCS Technique in Addition to Placement of a Cartilage Strut and Batten Grafts

Straight Rib for SEG Sutured to Caudal Septum & MCC

Fig. 12. Following transection of the LLCs, batten grafts are fixated to the newly rotated flap. The graft allows for reconstruction of the architecture of the lower nose. MCC, medial crural cartilage.

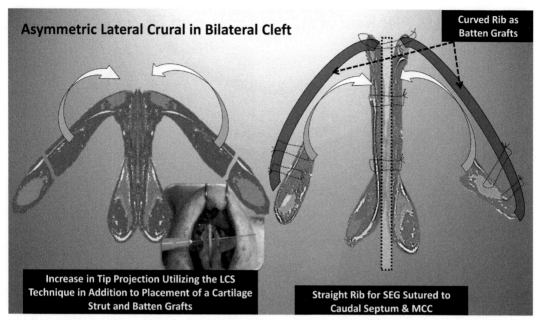

Fig. 13. In bilateral cleft cases, bilateral batten grafts are used to increase projection in conjunction with lateral crural rotational flaps. The batten grafts also fortify the lateral crus in the area of transection. MCC, medial crural cartilage.

starting from the piriform aperture and ending at the nasal bone suture line (at the level of the medial canthus)[1] (**Fig. 10**). The final step is creation of a greenstick fracture along the osteotomies with digital pressure to allow for mobilization of the lateral nasal walls and reduction of the nasal width.

Lower Lateral Cartilage, Batten Grafts, and the Nasal Tip

The LLC are the primary support structure for the nasal tip. In patients with cleft lip and palate, the LLC is collapsed vertically and positioned

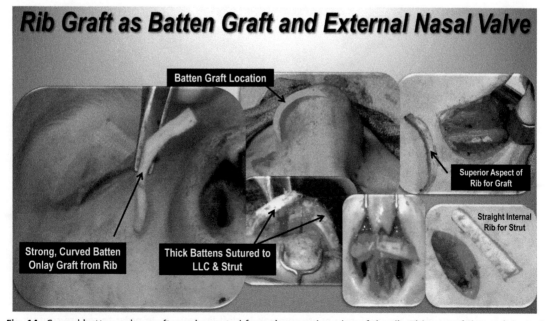

Fig. 14. Curved batten onlay grafts are harvested from the superior edge of the rib. This part of the graft is used to reconstruct the external nasal valve.

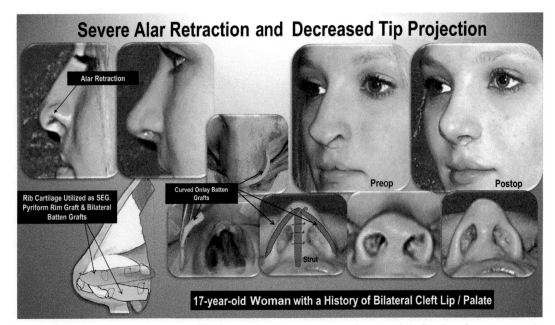

Fig. 15. Batten grafts play a pivotal role in treatment of alar retraction. The curved grafts allow for reconstruction of the alar base while assisting with nasal tip projection.

inferiorly, thus leading to an ill-defined tip contour. To properly address this deformity, the LLC must be identified and the number of available crus must be measured. A minimum of 5 to 7 mm of cartilage must be available for adequate tip support. If the width of the LLC is greater than 7 mm, a cephalic trim of the cartilage is performed to allow for proper rotation and positioning. Following the exposure of the LLC, the dome is exposed, and dissection continues until the

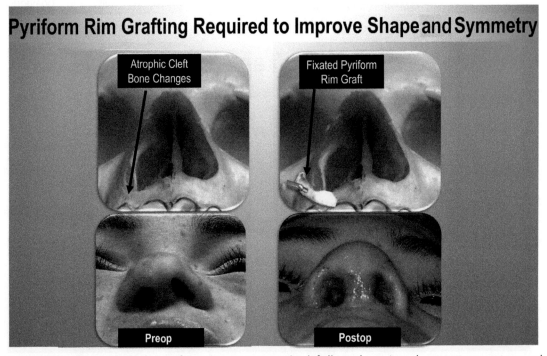

Fig. 16. Bony defects along the pyriform rim are common in cleft lip patients. In order to restore contour and symmetry, a graft is necessary to augment this region.

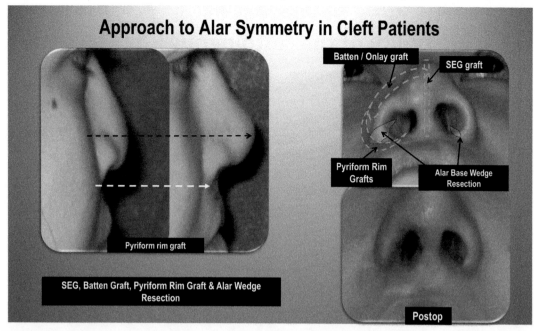

Fig. 17. Reconstruction of the pyriform rim involves the fixation of a cartilage graft to the bony defect. To achieve symmetry, an alar base wedge resection is required to establish comparable nasal openings.

septum is identified. At this time, the septum is addressed, and a portion of the septum may be harvested for fabrication of an SEG. The SEG is fixated to the caudal septum using 4-0 PDS sutures and then further immobilized by fixating the graft to the LLC, thus improving nasal tip projection and support (**Fig. 11**). The graft should be placed posterior and superior to the medial crura to avoid inadvertently widening the columella.[17] Fortification of the nasal base can be achieved by applying mattress sutures, allowing fixation of the medial crural cartilage to the septum

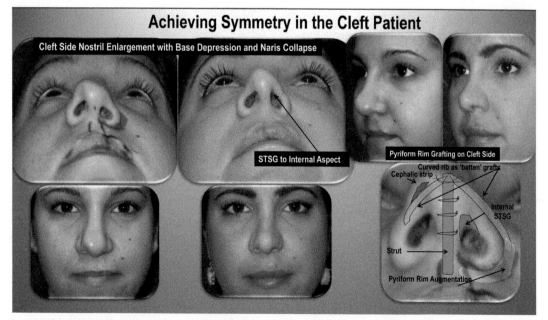

Fig. 18. Placement of a split-thickness skin graft (STSG) or composite graft along the internal aspect of the ala allows for an increase in the naris opening. Use of a graft improves symmetry between the nares and prevents nasal stenosis of the affected side. Placement of a pyriform rim graft demonstrates an elevation in the nasal base.

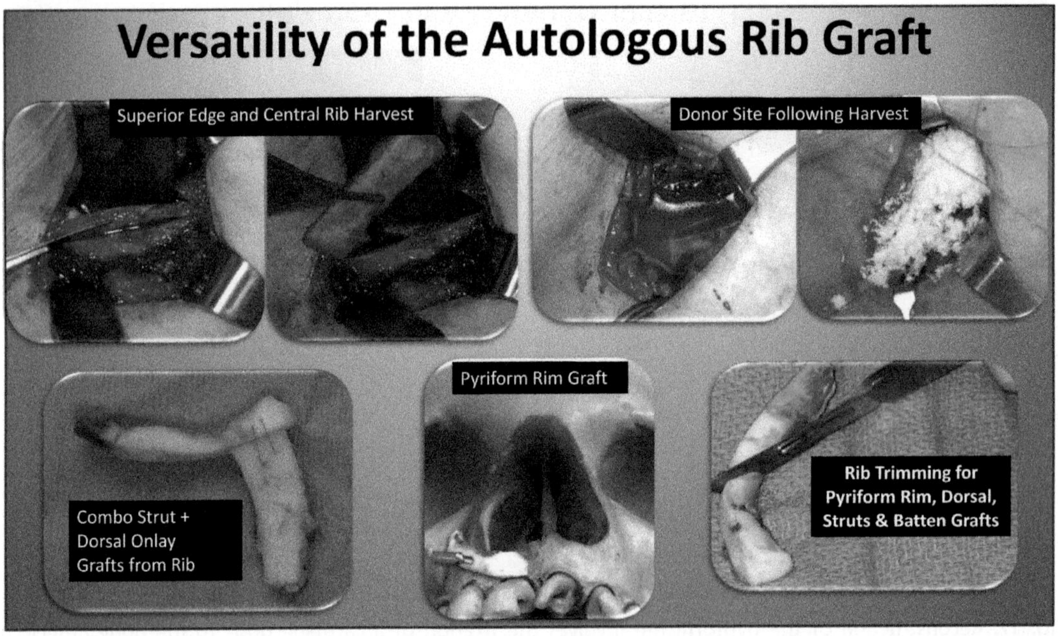

Fig. 19. Autologous rib cartilage is commonly harvested from the right sixth or seventh rib. A 5- to 6-cm segment is removed from the superior two-thirds of the medial cartilaginous rib. The inferior rib edge remains intact; this minimizes the surgical defect size and reduces postoperative pain.

and positioning the tip in a more cephalad position.[17] To achieve an improved contour to the nasal tip, a lateral crural steal (LCS) or advancement flap is implemented[2] (see **Figs. 4** and **5**). An LCS technique can be used in both unilateral and bilateral cleft lip and palate rhinoplasties. The LCS is achieved by increasing the length of the medial crura by sacrificing the length of the

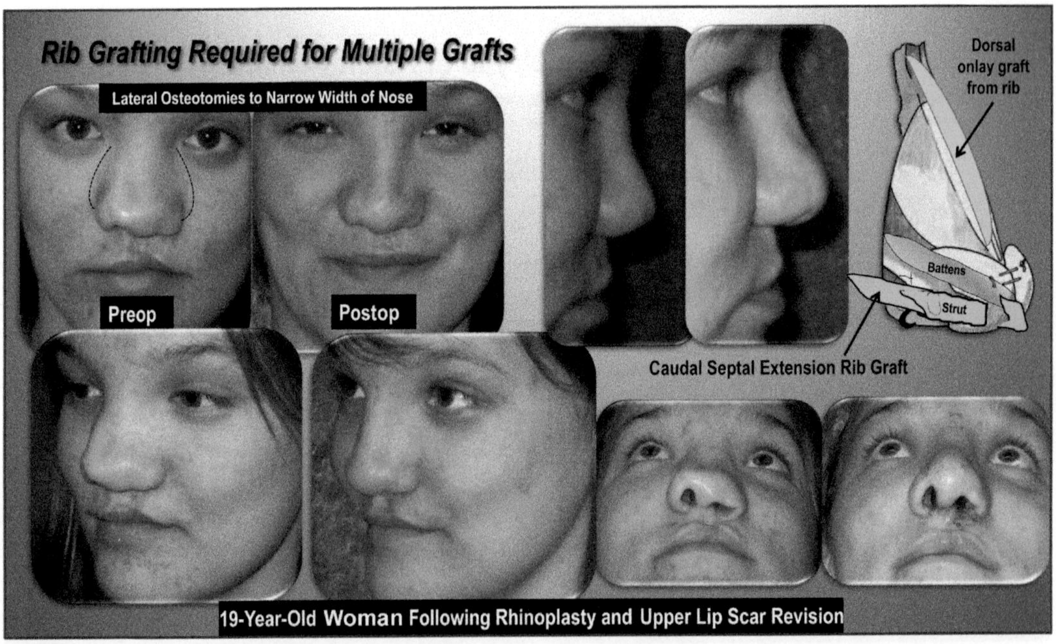

Fig. 20. Cleft lip and palate patients may require multiple grafts for nasal reconstruction. This patient required a dorsal onlay graft as well as batten, pyriform rim, and septal extension grafting. Before placement of a dorsal graft, lateral nasal bone osteotomies were performed in order to decrease the nasal width.

lateral crura. The lateral crura are advanced medially in a curvilinear manner to allow for the tip to be rotated superiorly and anteriorly, thus improving tip projection and symmetry (**Figs. 12** and **13**). Batten grafts fabricated from rib cartilage can be fixated to the LLC and SEG to create and strengthen a natural convex form of the external nasal valve[2] (**Fig. 14**). Batten grafts may be used to reconstruct a weakened LLC and play a pivotal role in the treatment of alar retractions (**Fig. 15**). To create excellent nasal tip projection and definition, 2 techniques can be applied: a shield graft and an SEG. A tip or shield graft may be placed between the junction of the intermediate and medial crura to further define the tip and increase projection. In addition to supporting the septum, SEG also provides excellent tip support. The graft should extend anteriorly past the septum approximately 4 to 5 mm with a thickness of at least 1 mm. It is recommended that these grafts be harvested from the rib cartilage because of the greater availability and quality of the cartilage as well as its ability to withstand postinflammatory changes.

Pyriform Rim and Premaxilla Augmentation

In addition to nasal structure deficiencies, cleft lip and palate patients may also present with bony deficits along the premaxilla, more specifically, the pyriform rim. Atrophic changes seen along

the pyriform rim cause an inferior and posterior displacement of the nose toward the cleft side. If during the rhinoplasty, the pyriform rim is not addressed, there will be continued asymmetric appearance of the nose, regardless if all other aspects of the surgery were well performed.[2] Several options are available to address this area. A rib graft, cortical bone graft, silicone implant, or even autologous fat grafting may augment the appearance of the pyriform[1] (**Fig. 16**).

Alar Base

The final step of the rhinoplasty is management of the alar base. The alar base on the cleft side can be found to be displaced inferiorly and laterally. Various surgical techniques may be implemented to rectify this displacement: V-Y advancement flap, sill resection, alar wedge resection (Weir procedure), and multiple suturing techniques. The authors use the Weir procedure to address the alar base because of its ability to manage excess lateral soft tissue and its open accessibility to the piriform rim for augmentation[2] (**Fig. 17**). A split-thickness skin graft or composite graft may be used in nostril enlargement in order to obtain symmetry (**Fig. 18**). Following alar reconstruction, a nostril retainer (Stryker Leibinger GmbH & Co, Freiburg, Germany) is recommended to assist with maintaining the contour of the naris.

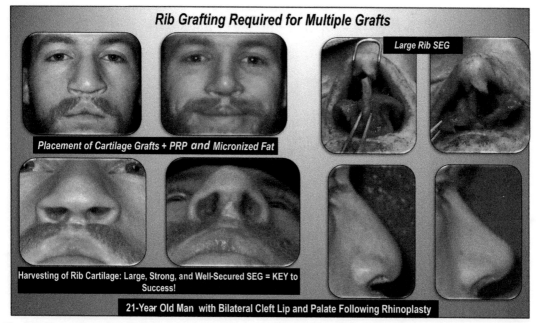

Fig. 21. The patient shown underwent augmentation with a cartilaginous rib graft, in the areas of the LLC and most importantly the caudal septum. The rib graft allows for a large and robust segment that functions as an SEG and assists with nasal projection. The patient underwent autologous fat grafting to recontour and restore the upper lip and philtrum shape, thus greatly improving the final results. PRP, platelet-rich plasma.

Autologous Rib Graft

In comparison to autologous grafts, alloplastic implants pose a greater risk for infection, dehiscence, and failure. For cleft lip and palate patients, the autologous rib graft is the primary choice for reconstruction of severe deformities, creation of nasal tip projection, and fortification of the underlying structures (**Fig. 19**). The rib graft is highly touted because of its quantity, resistance to scar contracture, overall strength, and versatility (**Figs. 20** and **21**). The major disadvantage of this graft is donor site morbidity, including postsurgical pain, scarring, and risk of a pneumothorax. When treating older cleft lip and palate patients with severe nasal deformities, the surgeon must be aware of possible ossification of the rib or even an increased incidence of graft warping.[2]

The autologous rib graft is harvested from the right sixth or seventh rib; the left ribs are avoided because of proximity to the heart. The harvesting technique begins with creating an incision with a number 10 blade over the selected rib. The dissection is carried out through the subcutaneous tissue and muscle using an electrocautery. Once the rib is encountered, an incision is made through the perichondrium. A subperichondral plane is developed and extends from the junction of the sternum and cartilage to the osseous-cartilaginous junction. A retractor is placed along the posterior aspect of the rib to protect the perichondrium as well as the lungs. Once the cartilage is harvested, it is imperative to evaluate for a possible pneumothorax. The surgical site is irrigated with saline, and positive pressure is applied to the lungs to assess for air leakage. The presence of any lung perforation must be addressed immediately. It is highly recommended to avoid full rib resection or discontinuous rib harvesting because of increased risk of postoperative complications.

Lip and Philtral Ridge

The use of fillers and autologous fat has provided the surgeon with a greater ability to address soft tissue deformities following a definitive rhinoplasty. The adjuvant therapies allow for enhancement of a deficient lip or philtral ridge on the cleft side, thus vastly improving the overall outcome. These therapies can greatly improve the overall results during rhinoplasty for the cleft lip and palate patient (**Figs. 22** and **23**). Synthetic filler and autologous fat can increase projection and restore volume to a flattened ridge or atrophic portion of the lip. Furthermore, fat grafting via micronized fat injection systems like ALMI provide the surgeon with the ability to restore lost volume and structural support. The presence of growth factors and preadipocytes allows for reduction of fibrosis along previous scar bands, thus improving the contour and texture of the scar (see **Fig. 21**).

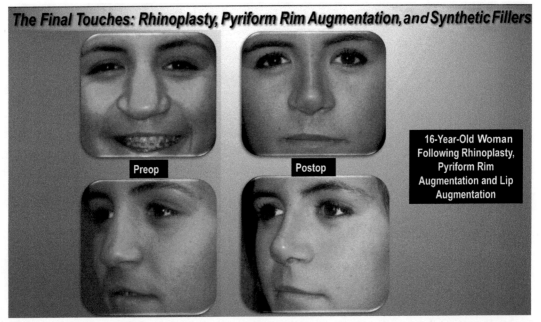

The Final Touches: Rhinoplasty, Pyriform Rim Augmentation, and Synthetic Fillers

Preop

Postop

16-Year-Old Woman Following Rhinoplasty, Pyriform Rim Augmentation and Lip Augmentation

Fig. 22. Bony defects along the pyriform rim and soft tissue defects along the upper lip can be addressed simultaneously during a rhinoplasty. The pyriform rim may be reconstructed with a cartilaginous graft while the upper lip can be treated with synthetic fillers. Treatment of these areas allows for improved esthetics following a rhinoplasty.

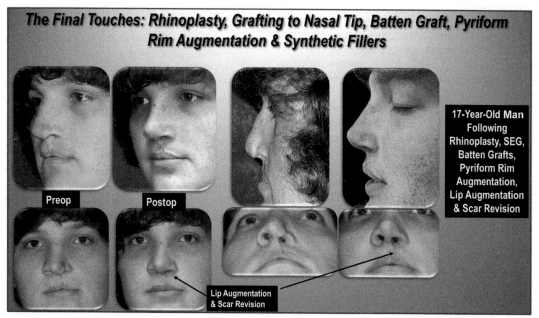

Fig. 23. This patient underwent reconstruction with multiple grafts, including an SEG, batten grafts, and pyriform rim grafts. The purpose of batten grafts is to rectify external valve collapse as well as treat alar retraction. Scar revision and lip augmentation play a key role in the overall esthetic outcome following a rhinoplasty.

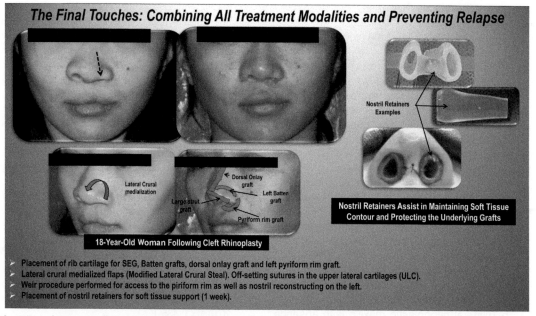

Fig. 24. A shorter medial crus and a longer lateral crus exist on the cleft side, resulting in a horizontally wider and displaced nostril on the cleft side, as shown. The patient underwent the classic grafting to the rim and tip as well as dorsal augmentation, which is more commonly required in the Asian cleft population. Nostril retainers are placed to assist with soft tissue contouring and support overlying grafts.

SUMMARY

Although cleft rhinoplasty is one of the most challenging and arduous procedures, the ability to improve the life of these patients is unremarkable. The results are both satisfying for the surgeon and life-changing for patients, as it provides symmetry, improved esthetics, and enhanced functionality. The depth of complexity originates from the requirement of multiple surgical stages over many years, involving numerous specialties.[20] The surgeon must have a thorough and complete understanding of the cleft anatomy while being able to assess both the esthetic and the functional limitations. Furthermore, the surgeon should be aware of various surgical techniques involving skin incisions, harvesting/grafting methods, framework reconstruction, and adjuvant therapies to achieve optimal esthetic and functional outcomes for patients (**Fig. 24**).

CLINICS CARE POINTS

- Secondary (definitive) rhinoplasty should be performed upon completion of facial growth and maturation. This occurs between the ages of 14-16 years in females and 16-18 years in males.
- Definitive rhinoplasty is performed once all skeletal discrepancies have been addressed.
- A majority of cleft lip and palate patients present with difficulty breathing due to severe septal deviation.
- Characteristics of unilateral cleft deformity:
  a Asymmetric tip
  b Posterior displacement of cleft-side dome
  c Deviation of the premaxilla, columella, and caudal nasal septum towards noncleft side
  d Alar base of the cleft side is positioned laterally, inferiorly, and posteriorly due to the pull of the orbicularis oris; widened ala
  e Cleft-side medial crus is blunted while lateral crus is elongated
  f Internal vestibular webbing along cleft side
  g As the caudal septum deviates toward the unaffected side, the remaining septum deviates toward the cleft side.
  h Anterior nasal spine is anterolaterally displaced
  i Maxillary hypoplasia along the cleft side
- Characteristics of bilateral cleft deformity:
  a More symmetrical deformity
  b Bilateral hypoplastic maxilla with absence of the nasal floor
  c Significant widening of the alar base with inferior and lateral positioning
  d Decreased projection and contour of the nasal tip
  e Bilateral elongated lateral crus and shortened medial crus
  f Bilateral vestibular webbing
- In order to increase the nasal tip projection, an asymmetric lateral crural steal technique must be combined with a septal extension graft as well as batten grafts.
- The autologous rib graft is harvested from the right side to avoid encountering the heart; the central portion of the rib is harvested to avoid warping.
- Autologous rib cartilage is utilized for septal extension, batten, and pyriform rim grafts.

DISCLOSURE

The authors have nothing to disclose.

REFERENCES

1. Kaufman Y, Buchanan EP, Wolfswinkel EM, et al. Cleft nasal deformity and rhinoplasty. Semin Plast Surg 2012;26(4):184–90.
2. Cuzalina A, Jung C. Rhinoplasty for the cleft lip and palate patient. Oral Maxillofac Surg North Am 2016; 28(2):189–202.
3. Gabriel, Martinez-Capoccioni and Carlos, Martin-Martin. Chapter 1: Cleft lip nasal deformity: analysis and treatment. Advances of Plastic and Reconstructive Surgery. Open Access Books. Available at: http://openaccessebooks.com/plastic-reconstructive-surgery/cleft-lip-nasal-deformity-analysis-and-treatment.pdf. Accessed August 25, 2018.
4. Baskaran M, et al. Cleft rhinoplasty. J Pharm Bioallied Sci 2015;2(suppl2):S691–4.
5. Sykes JM, Senders CW. Surgery of the cleft lip and nasal deformity. Oper Tech Otolaryngol Head Neck Surg 1990;1(4):219–24.
6. Berkowitz S. Lip and palate surgery. In: Berkowitz S, editor. Cleft lip and palate: diagnosis and management. New York: Springer; 2006. p. 315–51.
7. Slayer KE, et al. Unilateral cleft lip—approach and technique. Semin Plast Surg 2005;19(4):313–28.
8. Rossell-Perry P. Primary unilateral cleft lip nasal deformity repair using V-Y-Z plasty: an anthropometric study. Indian J Plast Surg 2017;50(2):180–6.
9. Subramanian CS, et al. A modified presurgical orthopedic (nasoalveolar molding) device in the treatment of unilateral cleft lip and palate. Eur J Dent 2016;10(3):435–8.
10. Jiri B, et al. Successful early neonatal repair of cleft lip within first 8 days of life. Int J Pediatr Otorhinolaryngol 2012;76(11):1616–26.

11. Massie JP, et al. Nasal septal anatomy in skeletally mature patients with cleft lip and palate. JAMA Facial Plast Surg 2016;18(5):347–53.

12. Good PM, Mulliken JB, Padwa BL. Frequency of Le Fort I osteotomy after repaired cleft lip and palate or cleft palate. Cleft Palate Craniofac J 2007;44(4): 396–401.

13. Petropoulos I, Karagiannidis K, Kontzoglou G. Our experience in open rhinoplasty. Hippokratia 2007; 11(1):35–8.

14. Koen JAOI, Orhan KS, van Heerbeek N. The effect of spreader grafts on nasal dorsal width in patients with nasal valve insufficiency. Arch Facial Plast Surg 2008;10(5):354–6.

15. Lee J-S, et al. March 24). Redefining the septal L-strut in septal surgery. PLoS One 2015. https://doi.org/10.1371/journal.pone.0119996.

16. Cerkes N. The crooked nose: principles of treatment. Aesthet Surg J 2011;31(Issue 2):241–57.

17. Guyuron B. MOC-PS(SM) CME article: late cleft lip nasal deformity. Plast Reconstr Surg 2008;121(4, Suppl):1–11.

18. Teymoortash A, Fasunla JA, Sazgar AA. The value of spreader grafts in rhinoplasty: a critical review. Eur Arch Otorhinolaryngol 2012;269(5):1411–6.

19. Saleh H, Khoury E. Closed rhinoplasty. In: Cheney ML, Hadlock TA, editors. Facial surgery: facial and reconstructive. Florida: CRC Press; 2015. p. 337–64.

20. Bendre DV1, Ofodile FA. Rhinoplasty in adolescent cleft patients. Oral Maxillofac Surg Clin North Am 2002;14(4):453–61.

Moving?

Make sure your subscription moves with you!

To notify us of your new address, find your **Clinics Account Number** (located on your mailing label above your name), and contact customer service at:

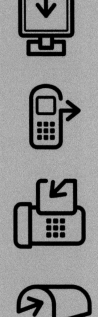

Email: journalscustomerservice-usa@elsevier.com

800-654-2452 (subscribers in the U.S. & Canada)
314-447-8871 (subscribers outside of the U.S. & Canada)

Fax number: 314-447-8029

Elsevier Health Sciences Division
Subscription Customer Service
3251 Riverport Lane
Maryland Heights, MO 63043